# Intermittent

# Fasting

## 2 Books in 1

by Rose Heale

*The Ultimate Way to Boost Your Metabolism and become Lean and Strong.*

*This book includes:*

**16/8 Intermittent Fasting**

*and*

**One Meal a Day**

Furthermore, the information that can be found within the pages described forthwith shall be considered both accurate and truthful when it comes to the recounting of facts. As such, any use, correct or incorrect, of the provided information will render the Publisher free of responsibility as to the actions taken outside of their direct purview. Regardless, there are zero scenarios where the original author or the Publisher can be deemed liable in any fashion for any damages or hardships that may result from any of the information discussed herein.

Additionally, the information in the following pages is intended only for informational purposes, and should thus be thought of as universal. As befitting its nature, it is presented without assurance regarding its prolonged validity or interim quality. Trademarks that are mentioned are done without written consent, and can in no way be considered an endorsement from the trademark holder.

# Table of Contents

# Book 1 : 16/8 Intermittent Fasting

by Rose Heale

*Gain Your Energy, Improve Your Mental Acuity, and Burn Fat Quickly; Become Healthy and Fit; The Most Complete Intermittent Fasting Book in 2019; Specifically for beginners.*

# Introduction

This book will help you in understanding the amazing concept of 16/8 Intermittent Fasting and the ways in which it can help you in your weight loss goals.

In the past few years, intermittent fasting has emerged as a new concept for weight loss that can fetch results. This book will explain the concept in detail, so that you can also take complete advantage of the process.

16/8 Intermittent fasting is a simple concept of following varied periods of feasting and fasting within the same day. However, the manner in which this needs to be done is very important.

Intermittent fasting is a concept that focuses less on what to eat, but emphasizes more on when to eat. It is a revolutionizing thought in an industry which has been obsessed with calories and lengthy diet preparations.

This book will explain the reasons the concept believes so and the scientific reasoning behind it. This book will also demonstrate the reasons which make the process highly effective and efficient.

This book will give you clear reasons for following intermittent fasting, and also the ways in which you can do so. It will show you the path to success in weight loss and explain the reasons due to which people fail in their attempts to lose weight.

It will guide you on the right path and show the common mistakes that can take you away from the path of success.

In an easy to understand manner, this book will provide all the information required to enable you to practice 16/8 intermittent fasting successfully.

There are plenty of books on this subject on the market, thanks again for choosing this one! Every effort was made to ensure it is full of as much useful information as possible. Please enjoy!

# Chapter 1: Can This Book Help You?

Have you been thinking, wishing, or praying to lose weight?

Do you dread the bulging fat tires?

Do you want to get rid of the saggy and sloppy physique, and convert it into a fit and lean shape?

Are you afraid of lifestyle disorders like diabetes, hypertension, heart problems, etc.? Are you serious about keeping them at bay?

Do you really, actually, and most definitely aspire for good health?

An affirmative answer means that this book can help you.

This is a book that will guide you towards good health in simple, effective, and actionable steps.

## Fun Fact

You would rarely find a person replying in negative to these questions. In fact, these have become some of the deepest yearnings of the current age.

You can find people ready to beg, borrow, or steal for the same if the results are a definite possibility.

However, it is also a stark reality that most people who aspire for these goals eventually end up failing. Not only this, most weight loss and wellness programs are never able to deliver on their promises of good health and weight loss.

The purpose of this book is not to demean other weight loss methods and lionize any one way to lose weight. This book will explain in plain and simple words the reasons for the failure of most weight loss methods, and the ways in which you can attain good health and lose weight.

This book will focus on the ways in which 16/8 Intermittent Fasting can help you in improving your overall health biomarkers, which would effortlessly lead to weight loss and fat burn.

The objective of this book is to explain two simple facts:

Weight loss is an achievable goal

Good health is not an anomaly, but a standard

Health issues are mostly a result of poor lifestyle and unhealthy choices we make in our eating habits and food items.

Therefore, if you follow some simple rules, both the goals of good health and weight loss are always within your reach for all intents and purposes.

Not only this, you can achieve them through most weight loss and fitness measures you might have followed till now.

However, tough routines, difficulties in making them a part of your daily routine, and unsustainability in long-term will lead to failure of any kind of weight loss measure.

This book will help you in finding, understanding, and following a weight loss and wellness measure that can help you in staying healthy and fit in long-term. It will help you in making a healthy routine a part of your lifestyle forever.

Long-Term **SUSTAINABILITY** is the central idea of this book. It will help you in understanding the ways through which you can make good health a part of your daily life, and weight loss would come naturally and effortlessly.

Therefore, the simple answer to the question is: **THIS BOOK WILL HELP YOU.**

If you want to know how, please stay with me throughout the book.

# Chapter 2: Tangible Goals You Can Achieve

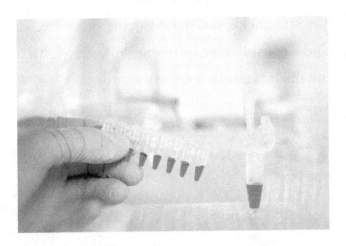

## Improvement in Overall Health Biomarkers

One of the biggest mistakes people often make is that they believe that once they lose weight, they will be able to work better on improving their health. If you are a proponent of this theory, then it is not going to take you anywhere. Weight gain is not the cause of the problem, but a consequence of poor health. If you are healthy and your body is functioning optimally, you would not accumulate excess weight in the first place.

The body has an exemplary process of balancing the energy reserves and expenditure through metabolic rate. Weight gain takes place when the body stops functioning at its optimal rate.

Intermittent fasting is a great way to improve overall health biomarkers. It is a routine through which you can help your body in course correction. Your body only needs a little support from you in optimizing the systems. Poor lifestyle, bad eating habits, and wrong food choices are responsible to a great extent for the health woes. Intermittent Fasting helps you in improving these areas steadily. You would find a considerable difference in your health once you start following the intermittent fasting routine.

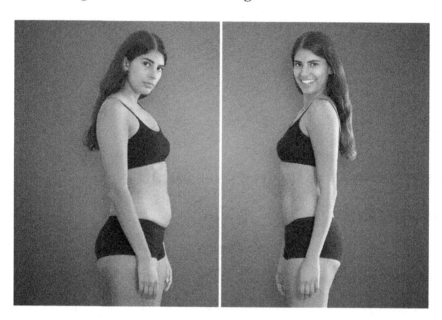

## Weight Loss

Obesity has started spreading its wings like an epidemic. More than 70% of the adult US population is either overweight or obese. This is a scary scenario. We all know that obesity is just not a cosmetic problem. It brings with itself a full package of issues. From metabolic disorders to health issues like diabetes and heart problems; the list is very long. The problem of obesity is well known, and people are trying their level best to get rid of the problem, but our more than four decades of a tryst with the problem and the offered solutions have made one fact very clear, it isn't easy to tackle.

Most weight loss measures are tough, painful, restricting, and extremely difficult to follow in long-term. Maintaining good health is not a one-time process. The process needs to be easy to follow and sustainable for it to work. From dieting to rigorous exercise routines, you can't follow a punishing routine endlessly, and that is the main cause of the problem.

Intermittent fasting is neither a diet nor does it involve punishing routines. It is a way to bring balance into your life. You can manage all facets of life effortlessly if you follow the routines. It is flexible, and you can always have the option to take things at your own pace.

It is a fact that intermittent fasting is no magical way to treat obesity. However, it is a healthy, safe, and sustainable way to bring down your weight and keep it under control in the long-term without having to put extra efforts continuously. To put it in simple words, intermittent fasting is a better way of life. By giving your body a fair chance to manage the energy accumulation and expenditure process, you are able to keep the weight under control very easily

.

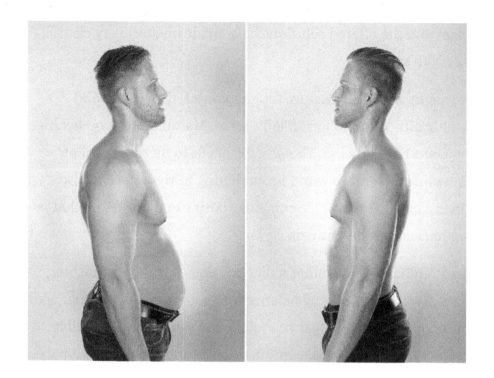

## Fat Burning

One of the biggest misconceptions created by the weight loss
industry is that fat burning and losing weight is the same thing.
Truth can't be farther from that. You can be losing weight without
burning even a gram of fat in your body, and that is not going to
help you at all. On the other hand, you may be burning a lot of fat.
However, your weight may not go down at all.

Weight loss and fat burn are two different things. When you are
burning fat and building muscles, your weight may not go down at
all. On the contrary, you may even notice a slight increase in your
weight while there would be a considerable reduction in your
waistline and fat deposits at your hips and thighs. In that case, you

would be making great progress as you would be losing dangerous visceral fat in your body, but building muscles at the same time. It means you would be getting healthier and stronger.

The muscles are compact but weigh more, while the fat is voluminous but weighs less. Therefore, even if you lose fat, you can gain weight. In that case, a slight increase in your weight wouldn't be a problem as your overall health would improve considerably, and you would lose the dangerous visceral fat at the same time.

Intermittent fasting has the ability to bring this positive change into your body. It creates the right conditions in your body, which allow the burning of fat and building of muscles. You will be able to burn your body fat faster than any other process as the main objective of the process is to initiate fat burning.

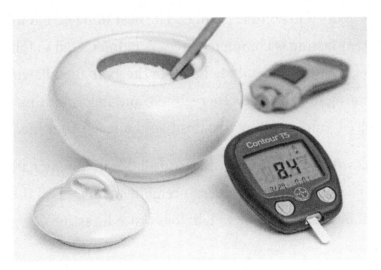

## Better Blood Sugar Management

Healthy management of blood sugar levels has emerged as a great challenge in the past few decades. It has become such a big problem that currently, more than 110 million people in the US alone are suffering from prediabetes and diabetes. Blood sugar spikes may not look like a very big problem, but they are the reason behind most health issues today. Consistently high blood sugar levels affect the healthy functioning of the vital organs, and also give rise to problems like hypertension, heart diseases, pancreatic issues, etc.

Intermittent fasting is one of the most reliable ways to manage high blood sugar levels safely. Your body gets the ability to manage the insulin levels better, and responds to it in a better way.

This book will help you in understanding the concept of intermittent fasting and the ways in which it can positively influence your body. It is an easy and effective way to manage your health as well as your weight and fat. It is easy to follow, and doesn't involve lengthy and complex things. The best thing is that following intermittent fasting is completely free. You don't need to follow costly diets or work for endless hours in the gym. By following a healthy eating routine, exercise regimen, and incorporating good food choices, you can bring this positive change in your life.

This book will show you the path to do all this in a sustainable manner, so that weight loss doesn't remain an on and off thing for you like it happens in other weight loss procedures.

# Chapter 3: The Real Problems in the path of Weight Loss

## Let There Be Light!

Once John came out of his home to find elderly Mr. Hobs looking frantically for something in his yard. Being a good Samaritan and a helpful neighbor, John asked Mr. Hobs what he was looking for. Mr. Hobs replied that he was unable to find his keys and was looking for them. John joined the search and started looking for the keys. After trying to find the keys in vain for a while, John asked the octogenarian neighbor if he remembered the place where he had placed the keys last. Mr. Hobs told that he remembered placing them somewhere inside the house. The enthusiasm for helping the elderly neighbor ended right away, and he wanted to know the reason behind the stupidity of looking for the keys outside when he remembered placing them last somewhere inside the house. Mr. Hobs curtly replied that the light was better outside.

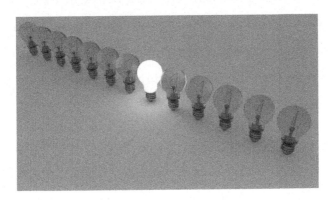

This might sound childish or stupid, but as far as the weight loss story goes, we are all walking down the same lines. We are looking for a solution in the wrong place. Most weight loss measures advocate a very simple concept that once your energy expenditure is higher than your energy consumption, you would start losing weight. The way to reduce the energy intake is to lower your calorie intake, and that should solve the problems for you.

This idea may look like an ideal solution, but sadly, it isn't.

We consider our body to be a machine, but don't give it the due credit of intelligence. We expect more intelligence from our electronic devices, but fail to appreciate the intelligence each cell in our body carries. Our body has been through millions of years of evolution. It is designed to survive in the toughest times. We have survived the dark ages. We have been through the toughest floods and famines. We have thrived in spite of the fact that we are among the weakest of the prey. Without long claws, big teeth, or enormous weight, our ancestors have hunted lions, bears, and elephants. We are nowhere even close to being the fastest or even fast enough, and yet with basic means, we have outrun everything on this blue planet. It all happened because our body learned and kept adapting continuously.

Storing fat has always been part of the survival mechanism. The body stores fat so that in times of extreme calorie deficit, it can be used to prolong survival till the energy supply resumes. Not only humans, but most animals on this planet have this mechanism inbuilt. It has worked wonderfully for everyone on this globe except humans as seen in the past few decades. The boon for survival has become a bane. However, it is surprising that any other undomesticated animal species on the planet is not facing the obesity epidemic.

The fat storage mechanism is perfect, and is not at fault. It is the way our eating habits, lifestyle, and food choices have changed that is making the difference.

# Ambiguities in the Theory of Bringing Weight Loss through Calorie Deficit

Our body has a mechanism to judge the calorie intake deficit, and it can and will adjust itself to manage it. Simply reducing the calorie intake cannot be the solution to the problem as advertised so hawkishly by the weight loss industry.

## *The Basic Idea*

Our body needs energy continuously for running the physical processes. Breathing, blood circulation, perspiration, temperature control, and hundreds and thousands of processes going on inside the body need continuous energy supply. These are the metabolic functions. Your body needs a certain number of calories every day to run these functions. You would need these many calories even if you don't do any other kind of physical activity.

This is called the **Basal Metabolic Rate** (BMR)

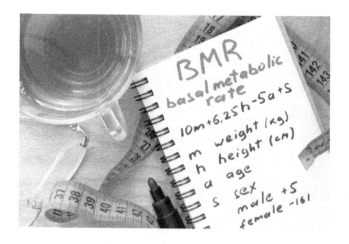

If you do any kind of physical activity like running, walking, intense exercise or even going to the office and sitting for the whole day at your desk, it would mean that you would also need some additional calories for carrying out these functions.

People with an active lifestyle would need more calories, and people with a more sedentary lifestyle would have lower energy demand.

Some weight loss experts believe that by simply lowering the calorie intake, they can force the body to start burning the fat reserves. They believe that simple calorie restriction can be an ideal way to bring weight loss.

## The Problem With the Idea

Once you get on any kind of weight loss diet, the first thing you do is reduce your calorie intake. This means if your daily calorie requirement is 2000, you can reduce weight by consuming only 1500 calories a day. Your body will have no other option than to fulfill the deficit of 500 calories from your body fat. This deficit of 500 calories is the key to weight loss.

If you have been led into believing that then you have been seriously wronged, once you start reducing the daily calorie intake by 500 calories, your body will take it as a scarcity of food. Your existence and knowledge may be only a few decades old, but the evolutionary knowledge stored in the cells is of millions of years. It has the knowledge and experience of dealing with such scarcities, and knows the ways to manage them. The first thing the body would do is lower the metabolic rate to manage the calorie deficit.

This means that your body would start by managing energy expenditure process. It would drop the metabolic rate, and you would start feeling lethargic, lazy, dull, and weak. Doing any kind of physical activity requires energy expenditure, and your body is trying to save energy to buy as much time as possible until the regular energy supply is restored.

The second thing it does is to dump the excess water from your body. The excess water, apart from providing hydration also helps in maintaining body temperature. It means it helps in keeping the body cool in summers and warm in winters. It keeps you comfortable in all weathers. However, when the body needs to choose between comfort and survival, it would always go for the latter. When following restrictive calorie diets, you would feel that your tolerance for the weather goes down. You start feeling colder or warmer.

When the body dumps a lot of water, it leads to a weight loss effect, as water has considerable weight. However, this is a temporary phenomenon because as soon as you would start eating normally or your body gets adjusted to the calorie deficit diet, the water weight would come back again. This small victory is often short-lived.

The people who think that they can burn a lot of calories by lifting weights in the gym for hours are also misled. There is no doubt in the fact that when you work out in the gym for long, your energy expenditure increases. It means you really start burning calories. If you are consuming 2000 calories a day, but follow a workout routine that involves burning 1000 extra calories apart from the ones your body is burning in running the metabolic functions, you would certainly lose weight. However, there are two major problems in this process.

i.      **For how long can you sustain this routine**

It is not unusual for people to get inspired to lose weight and head to the gym. In the beginning, enthusiasm is high, and people give more than their best. They work hard, and sometimes go beyond their physical limits.

However, spending long hours in the gym can make you exert force. Apart from losing weight, people also have to do other things like earn money, maintain balance in personal and professional life.

This enthusiasm generally doesn't last very long, and then the laid-back attitude takes over the resolve. It is not about determination, but the practicality of life. For most of us, it isn't possible to lift weights in the gym for hours in the morning and evening, and then lead a highly professional life with cut-throat competition and no capping on working hours. This is a reason why workout routines don't last very long for most people.

ii. **Imbalance in Diet**

When people begin high-intensity workouts, they also need to increase their calorie intake. It might come in the form of high protein intake or consuming a more nutrient dense diet. The problem is that although people start reducing the time devoted to exercise over time, the calorie intake remains the same, and it also leads to weight gain. The body gets into the mode where the energy needs to increase substantially, but the expenditure goes down gradually.

Although exercise is a great way to lose weight, it usually proves to be ineffective for most people due to the two reasons mentioned above.

It is important that you understand that the calorie calculation is not that simple. You simply cannot force your body to start burning the stored calories because you have reduced the calorie intake. The body always thinks about survival in the long-term. It has evolved that way. There are some important things for you to understand.

## Fat Is Not a Villain

Your body doesn't consider fat to be an existential threat. On the contrary, fat serves several crucial functions. It is the building base for the most important hormones in the body. It is the energy reserve your body keeps for rainy days when there would be an acute shortage of energy supply. Your body can easily start using fat for producing energy when really needed. The energy produced by burning fat is not only high in potency, but also releases less waste. Therefore, the body loves to accumulate fat. Fat in the body also provides insulation against cold temperatures.

Your body likes to store fat. For it, fat is a good thing. The problem begins when the storage of fat goes out of hand. Excess of even the most wonderful things can mean trouble.

When your body starts accumulating excess fat, most of the processes that control the body go flat. This leads to a serious imbalance, and that eventually leads to problems. Therefore, simply branding fat as the main problem and ignoring the issues that lead to an imbalance in fat accumulation would be a poor strategy.

The real problem is the imbalance that leads to the accumulation of excess fat in the body. Once you are able to understand the reasons behind the problem, fighting it would become easier.

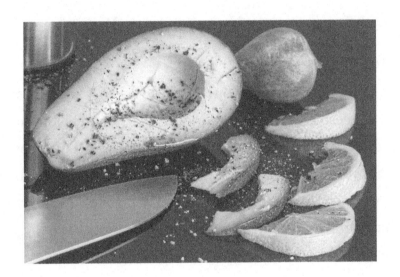

# Chapter 4: Insulin Resistance— The Real Culprit

Insulin is not a word that you may not have heard before. The pancreas in the body releases the insulin hormone. It plays several crucial functions in your body.

## Three Main Functions of Insulin

### Absorption of Glucose

Whenever you eat anything, your body processes it and turns it into glucose. Glucose is the simplest form of energy, and all the cells in your body can directly use it for producing energy. The glucose mixes into your bloodstream and raises the blood sugar level. As soon as the blood sugar level rises, the pancreas senses it and starts releasing insulin to stabilize the blood sugar level, as very high blood sugar level can be dangerous in the long run.

The cells can directly use glucose for producing energy, but they need insulin to help them absorb glucose. Therefore, insulin acts as the passkey. It attaches itself to the cells, and they can absorb as much glucose as they require. Without the help of insulin, the cells in your body cannot absorb glucose, and they'd starve to death. This would eventually mean that even you can't survive without insulin.

## Blood Sugar Level Stabilization

Another function of insulin is to lower blood glucose levels. The cells have a limited capacity to absorb glucose, as they can't store much. Therefore, all the excess glucose will remain in the bloodstream as blood glucose. However, high blood glucose can be dangerous, as it would start hardening the arteries and also affect the functioning of the vital organs like heart, kidneys, and liver. This is the reason why people with poor blood sugar control are generally at high risk of multiple organ failure.

Your pancreas keeps pumping insulin till the time blood sugar levels in your blood get low. Once your cells stop absorbing glucose, the insulin gets on the process of storing the glucose in other forms in various parts of the body. First, it stores the glucose as glycogen in the muscles and liver, and the remaining glucose is stored as fat in the fat cells.

## Fat Storage

Fat storage is the main task of insulin hormone. It is the master fat storage hormone in your body. It means that your fat cells are under the direct command of insulin. As long as insulin levels in your blood are high, your body would remain in fat storage mode. This also means that if the insulin levels in your blood are high, no matter what you do, your body will not start burning stored fat. You must understand very clearly that fat storage and fat burning are two contradictory processes, and can't go side by side.

## Now Let's Understand the Fat Storage Process Clearly

Whenever you eat anything, that has calories; even a sip of soda, even the diet soda or zero calorie soda comes under this category.

- ✓ Eating or drinking anything with calories will lead to the release of glucose in the bloodstream.
- ✓ This would spike your blood sugar levels.
- ✓ To stabilize the blood sugar levels, the pancreas would release insulin.
- ✓ Once released, it takes anywhere between 8-12 hours for the insulin levels to go down in your bloodstream.
- ✓ This means that after your last meal, your body would need minimum 8-12 hours before it can begin the fat burning process.
- ✓ If you have a habit of frequent snacking, late night eating, drinking soda or other sweetened beverages like tea, coffee, shakes, etc. at short intervals, then your blood sugar levels would remain consistently high. This would also mean that the insulin levels in your blood would also remain consistently high.
- ✓ When the insulin levels in the blood remain perennially high, the cells become less sensitive or unresponsive to the insulin signals.

- ✓ This means that although there may be a high presence of insulin in your blood, it may not be able to attach itself to the cells to facilitate glucose absorption.
- ✓ This would also mean that your blood sugar levels would remain high for unusually longer.
- ✓ The pancreas will sense this, and it would frantically keep pumping more and more insulin into your bloodstream to stabilize the blood sugar levels at the earliest.
- ✓ This even aggravates the problem in place of reducing it. Higher insulin presence in the bloodstream would mean slower reaction of the cells.
- ✓ It would also mean that your body would take even much longer to get into the fat burning mode, and the insulin would be present for a longer duration due to its high presence.
- ✓ In case of densely populated developed countries like the US, their bodies experience high insulin presence all the time. They never abstain from consuming calories for long periods which the insulin levels can dissipate.
- ✓ Such people cannot experience fat burn at all, no matter how many calorie restrictive diets they follow.
- ✓ A consistently high blood sugar level also forces the pancreas to keep working. This leads to fatigue in this important and sensitive organ, which may result in pancreatic problems.
- ✓ The real problem remains that as long as insulin levels are high in your body, no matter how much effort you put into burning fat, it is not going to happen.

Simply put, consider insulin as the commanding officer of the army. As long as the commanding officer is standing, the troops can't relax. They will have to remain in an attention pose, and this is the main problem.

If you seriously and sincerely want to lose weight, the only way to achieve is to get around this insulin problem.

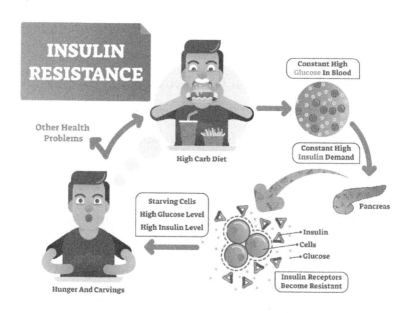

## The Phenomenon of Insulin Resistance

Insulin resistance is a state in which your cells become so overexposed to the insulin that they stop responding curtly to the insulin signals.

It is a very common thing to happen if you have a habit of frequent snacking. Most of us don't realize, but frequent snacking can cause greater harm than not eating for a few days at all.

The quantity of food you are eating becomes immaterial in this scenario, as it is not about storing more fat, but about burning the stored fat. To burn even a gram of fat in the body, first, it will have to get out of the fat storage mode, and that can't happen as long as insulin is present in the bloodstream in high quantity.

This overexposure of insulin to the cells is termed as **Insulin Resistance**. If a person is suffering from insulin resistance, then it is the base of all the problems.

This book will focus mainly on this problem, and the ways to bring your body out of continuous fat storage mode. It isn't a very complicated thing to do, but requires some specific conditions for that to take place. Ignoring this part leads to the failure of most weight loss strategies. If there is some amount of fat loss, it is very quick to come back again.

If you also believe that weight relapse is a never-ending problem, then intermittent fasting can put a full stop on all your worries once and for all. Intermittent fasting is a reliable way to lower the weight and manage it successfully.

Intermittent fasting is not only a reliable way to reverse insulin resistance, but the **MOST EFFECTIVE WAY** to bring reverse **INSULIN RESISTANCE**.

# Chapter 5: Reasons Behind Increasing Insulin Resistance in People

## Let's Begin With Some Facts

One-third of the US population is currently suffering from diabetes or prediabetes. This means that the next person you might meet after reading this book can be suffering from this problem. However, that is not even close to scary. Stats show that more than 110 million people in the US are affected by prediabetes and diabetes. Out of these, around 30 million people have diabetes. They know about the problem and are taking medication to manage their blood sugar levels. However, approximately 84 million people currently suffering from prediabetes may not even know that they have a problem.

Diabetes is a silent killer. A person developing prediabetes may not have symptoms for decades. However, this doesn't reduce the risk; in fact, it increases the risk greatly. Diabetes and prediabetes are mainly lifestyle disorders. It means that a person suffering from these issues and not paying attention to them will become prone to greater problems.

A person suffering from prediabetes will not need insulin, or any other medication for decades. But this doesn't mean that it isn't causing damage. Prediabetes is a major cause of chronic kidney disease (CKD). Here, it is important to acknowledge the fact that CKD is the 8 biggest cause of deaths in the US. Prediabetes keeps putting the load on the kidneys. It also keeps increasing the blood pressure levels slowly, and all these things eventually lead to kidney damage.

Even scarier is the fact that a person suffering from prediabetes may have normal blood sugar results on random testing. The reliable way to detect prediabetes is to take hbA1C or A-One-C test. This test determines the mean blood sugar levels of the past three months.

Prediabetes can go undetected and symptomless for decades. There are some very common symptoms like increased thirst and hunger, food cravings, dry mouth, frequent urination, and urinary infections. Some people can also experience unexplained weight loss, fatigue, headaches, blurred vision, etc.

However, if you look at the rate at which people are affected by this problem, it is always wise to take proper tests, so that this problem can be nipped in the bud.

# The Prime Reason for Prediabetes is Insulin Resistance

Prediabetes happens when the blood sugar levels start remaining high in your body. This can only happen when the insulin in your body is not able to lower the blood sugar levels quickly and properly. The longer the blood sugar levels remain high, the higher the chances of prediabetes for you.

This only happens when your cells start developing insulin resistance. The slower they respond to the insulin signals, the longer it would take to stabilize the blood sugar levels. In the meantime, the pancreas would keep pumping more and more insulin to facilitate faster absorption of blood sugar. It starts a vicious cycle that leads to insulin resistance, prediabetes, and eventually, diabetes.

# The Causes of the Development of Insulin Resistance

The main reason for the development of insulin resistance in the body is a frequent insulin spike. To understand this clearly, let's revisit the process once again.

Blood Sugar Management in a Healthy Individual Works as Follows:

Calorie Intake

Glucose Release-
Increase in Blood
Sugar Levels

Pancreas Pumps
Insulin to Lower
Blood Sugar

Insulin Binds itself to
the cells and
facilitates glucose
absorption

Blood sugar levels go
down

However, it works differently in case of people suffering from insulin resistance:

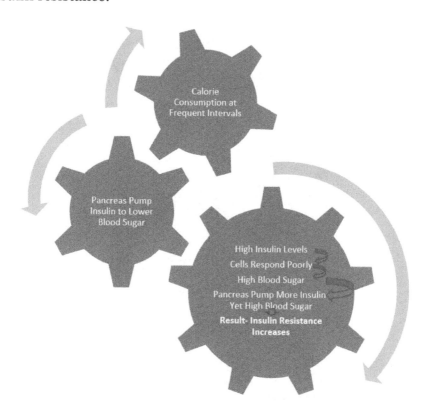

If a person develops insulin resistance, the process; which is designed to lower the blood sugar levels, starts working against it.

The main cause of insulin resistance is the high presence of prolonged exposure of insulin to the cells.

# Ways to Prevent Prolonged Insulin Exposure

The simple answer to this is by reducing the instances of an insulin spike in the body. This is simple, yet the most effective way to not only bring down insulin resistance, but also lower the risk of prediabetes and diabetes. It will also help you in fighting obesity, and we will go to that in detail.

As we have already discussed, the consumption of calories in any form would lead to an insulin spike in our body.

- This means that whenever you eat or drink anything that has calories, it will lead to the release of glucose in your blood.
- The blood sugar levels would rise.
- Your pancreas will pump insulin to lower the blood sugar levels. This would create an insulin spike.
- The insulin levels would slowly recede within 8-12 after your last meal.
- If you consume anything within this time, there would be again an insulin spike and the clock of 8-12 hours would get reset.
- The insulin levels would remain high in your blood without a break, and you will remain at risk of developing insulin resistance.
- This problem would eventually lead to prediabetes and diabetes later on.

Now, simply run this scenario in your mind and think about your routine or the routine of people around you. It won't be surprising if you find more than a dozen people ignorantly falling in the trap of prediabetes.

Our lifestyles have become such that we have become habitual of frequent snacking. We never give a second thought to the glass of soda, tea, coffee, chewing gum, munchies, coming in front of us.

## Poor Eating Habits; the Main Cause of the Problem

When it comes to obesity, diabetes, and other lifestyle disorders, sugar and unhealthy food items are the usual suspects. There is no denying the fact that they play a very important role in causing the problem, but they didn't cause the problem in the first place.

Your body has the processes to process sugar. It does put an extra load on your liver and the body, and produces a lot of toxins. If your eating habits are in control, and you are not yet suffering from diabetes, moderate consumption of sugar wouldn't cause much damage.

Here, it is important to understand that I am not advocating or encouraging the consumption of sugar. I just want to highlight the fact that we have been looking for the problem where it doesn't exist. The real problem is not in the consumption of sugar, fried food, fast food, or street food.

The problem is in consuming food too often. The real problem is with frequent snacking. The problem is in following an unregulated, unrestricted, and undisciplined eating routine.

Even if you are eating the healthiest food items 8 times a day, it would cause insulin spikes in your blood and eventually insulin resistance.

The food industry has pushed the idea of small but frequent meals into our heads. It has its vested interests. The food joints profit from your habit of eating on temptation. However, that neither makes it safe nor healthy.

The only way to prevent prediabetes is to develop insulin sensitivity. That can only happen when the insulin levels in your body would start remaining low for a considerable period within every day.

Intermittent Fasting is the only way to do it. It will not only help in reversing insulin resistance, but will also help in developing insulin sensitivity in the body.

In the following chapters, we will understand in detail the ways in which intermittent fasting can help you in these problems, and how that would lead to weight loss, fat burn and improvement in overall health biomarkers.

# Chapter 6: What Is Intermittent Fasting?

Put in simple terms; intermittent fasting is sporadic eating. It is a lifestyle in which you will have to follow an eating pattern which will have longer fasting windows and shorter feasting windows within the same day.

Some people start feeling intimidated by the term 'fasting', as that usually means leaving food for prolonged durations. In principle, intermittent fasting is also the same. However, the fasting duration is generally not very long, and the fasting lasts only a few hours every day. This is the reason that makes it **ACTIONABLE** and **SUSTAINABLE**.

We divide intermittent fasting into two parts:

**Fasting Window:**

- This the duration in which you will remain in a complete fasted state.
- This duration will be comparatively longer than the fasting window.
- You cannot eat or drink anything that has calories.
- Only some beverages like water, unsweetened fresh lime, unsweetened black tea, and coffee can be consumed during this period.

## Feasting Window:

- This is the period in which you can consume your meals.
- You will need to divide your complete nutrition in two-three fulfilling meals.
- You will have to get rid of the habit of snacking, eating, and drinking very often.
- There will be no restriction on the number of calories you can consume in your meals.
- You can consume a reasonable amount of food in this duration as per your physical needs.

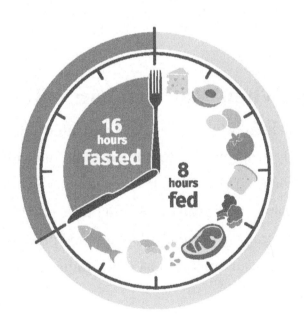

# Intermittent Fasting Isn't a Diet

The first and foremost thing that you must clear in your mind is that intermittent fasting isn't a diet. It is a way of life. It is a way to improve your eating habits and bring a positive change to your system. Intermittent fasting helps in balancing the physical processes inside your body. It is a way to manage the overworked systems and give them the required rest. To do all this, you don't need to do anything extra. You only need to abstain from doing anything extra.

It means it doesn't require lengthy food preparations. There will be no need for lengthy food charts. It is a process to bring harmony inside your body.

# Focus on 'When' Rather Than 'What'

The substantial difference between diets and intermittent fasting is that diets mostly focus on what to eat. However, intermittent fasting has its focus on when to eat. When we started our journey as complex organisms on this earth, we didn't have much choice over food. There are organs in our body that are used process grass and cellulose. Our body can process most of the things if consumed in moderate quantities.

Intermittent fasting puts its complete focus on the timing of eating, and hence the 'when' is very important in it. You will have to follow the feasting and fasting windows sincerely and religiously. It is the only thing that is going to make all the difference.

Intermittent fasting helps in improving

a. Insulin sensitivity
b. Brings better satiety control (Leptin sensitivity)
c. Lowers free fatty acids
d. Brings down chronic inflammation
e. Initiates fat burning
f. Reduces the risk of heart diseases
g. Helps in better management of hypertension

All these things eventually lead to good health. When your body becomes healthy, and all the vital functions start functioning smoothly, the body doesn't feel the need to hoard fat. In fact, the fat burning mechanism becomes smooth, and you start burning healthily.

All this can happen once you start emphasizing on the 'when' aspect of eating.

## It is Liberating

People all over the globe loath the process of weight loss more than their weight. This happens even though the excess weight can kill them due to its harmful impact on the body. Yet, people despise weight loss measures. The reason behind this detestation is simple; most weight loss measures are restricting, frustrating, punishingly painful, and tough. Weight gain is involuntary, but the process to get is off is mercilessly painful.

Either you follow a diet or strict exercise routines, they both drain the practitioners, which is a necessity.

One of the best things about intermittent fasting is that it isn't a punishing routine. There is no doubt that you wouldn't get a free ride. There would be rules. There would be some restrictions. However, intermittent fasting can be easily incorporated into the lifestyle, and hence, after a while, you stop feeling the pinch. You need to have moderate control over your eating habits and food choices. No food item is completely prohibited, and hence, there is generally no temptation building. You'd mostly remain free to eat anything you like in a moderate quantity.

## It is Easy to Follow

The only strict requirement in intermittent fasting is to maintain steady fasting and feasting routine. It means that you will have to maintain certain numbers of fasting hours every day. However, it doesn't remain a challenge as you would be doing it on a daily basis. It becomes a part of your life. Managing those hours is generally effortless.

Usually, the shorter intermittent fasting routines last 14-16 hours. A large portion of this time is spent sleeping, and hence, you only experience fasting for a short duration. The hunger pangs may trouble you for a couple of days in the beginning, but they never remain a permanent problem. Within a few days of following the routine, you would not need to do anything extra to manage the routine.

## You Don't Need to Go an Extra Mile

One of the biggest problems with weight loss measures is that they are not only difficult, but costly and cumbersome. They require lengthy planning and preparation. Intermittent fasting requires nothing of that sort. It is not about anything extra in your routine, but about removing extra things from daily life. In fact, following intermittent fasting can be cost effective for you. It eliminates most of the snacks and beverages from your routine, and hence, you'd be able to save a lot of money.

The focus of intermittent fasting is to give your blood sugar management process the required rest. It also helps in providing the much-needed respite to your gut. Your body is able to process the nutrients better, and hence, you would feel healthier and better.

# Chapter 7: Various Intermittent Fasting Protocols

Fasting of any form requires discipline. You will have to exercise a considerable amount of self-control. People who have undertaken any type of diet would be able to understand this easily. However, I'd like to say that intermittent fasting doesn't even come half-way in comparison to restrictive calorie diets in the difficulty level.

Therefore, if you have been perspiring while thinking about the ordeals that you might have to undertake to give another attempt to weight loss, you can simply relax. Intermittent fasting is easy and becomes effortless after a while.

## The Rules

1. You can't eat anything during the fasting window.
2. You can't have frequent snacks and beverages even during your eating window.
3. You can eat anything healthy in moderate quantity during the eating window.

These are the simple rules of intermittent fasting that you would need to follow.

Intermittent fasting doesn't put too many restrictions on you, and that's what makes it so easy to follow.

Types of Intermittent Fasting Protocols

There are several intermittent Fasting protocols that you can follow. As the protocol changes, the number of fasting and eating hours change.

Some Major Intermittent Fasting Protocols are:

## 12/12 Intermittent Fasting Protocol

This is the easiest intermittent fasting protocol to begin with. The process is very simple; you need to remain in the fasted state for 12 hours, and eat healthily during the remaining 12 hours. The actual of this intermittent fasting protocol is to slowly develop self-control over eating habits and extend the fasting hours. It is very easy to follow as you can simply choose the 12 hours of the night for your fasting window. It is not only easy, but even preferable. Your body starts getting the time to process all the energy consumed during the day. The 12-hour eating window needs to be used for having 3 meals a day. These three meals would be the only way of consuming calories. You should use this routine to learn ways to eliminate the habit of snacking completely from your life.

This is simply an initiation technique, and once you get used to 12 hours fasting, you can move to the next intermittent fasting protocol, i.e., the 16/8 Intermittent Fasting Protocol.

## 16/8 Intermittent Fasting Protocol

This is the most popular and successful intermittent fasting protocol. It requires you to maintain a fasting window of 16 hours a day, and eat within the 8 hours of eating window. The reason behind the success of this intermittent fasting protocol is its long-term sustainability. It is so easy to follow that you can continue with this routine effortlessly without having to think about it. This means that you can follow it for years without having to take a break. This intermittent fasting protocol not only helps you in losing weight and burning fat, but it is also very helpful in gaining muscles at the same time. Following it even ensures that weight relapse doesn't take place at all.

A little modification in this intermittent fasting protocol known as 14/10 is considered ideal for women. This is a bit easier and equally beneficial for women. Fasting for 14 hours and maintaining a healthy lifestyle in the 10 hours eating window can help women not only in losing the extra pounds, but would also give them great health benefits.

You can follow this intermittent fasting protocol irrespective of the line of business you follow or kind of lifestyle you have. Even the people in the food industry can follow this intermittent fasting protocol. People following diets find it very difficult to work in the food industry as working at places where all kinds of food items are present makes it very difficult for them to control the urge to eat. With intermittent fasting, there would be no such problem. You will have a healthy eating window in which you can eat whatever you wish to eat within reasonable limits. This intermittent fasting protocol makes it guilt-free. You don't have to always  keep making a choice between the devil and the deep blue sea. It would never make food your enemy.

It is inclusive, easy to follow, and a very balanced way to live a healthy life. A healthy diet and exercise routine can make losing weight even faster and easier with this routine.

**20/4 Intermittent Fasting Protocol**

This intermittent fasting protocol requires you to fast for 20 hours a day and eat within the remaining 4 hours of eating window. It is a tough routine to maintain, and is suitable only for people who have strict muscle gain goals. This is a routine for bodybuilders and people going for performance enhancement. Sportsmen and athletes follow this routine as it helps in increasing the production of some hormones that give a great boost to their stamina

Undoubtedly, this is a tough routine. The four-hour eating window can be used for having two meals; one meal being smaller and other being the complete meal. However, it is not a sustainable routine as fasting for 20 hours is always difficult, and the body never really gets used to the routine. A person following this routine would have the hunger pangs at the end of the routine.

# One-Meal-a-Day Fasting Diet

One Meal a Day goes one step ahead of the previous routine. The fasting hours increase to 23 hours, and you only get one hour to have your meals. It may look like a punishing routine, but people follow this routine with great success. Like in the case of the previous routine, the body can never really get used to 23 hours of fasting. Therefore, hunger pangs would always be felt around the end of the fasting routine. However, they don't remain such a big problem as you would be experiencing them for a while daily.

On the other hand, the positive health impact of the routine is tremendous. This routine can prove to be a key to eliminate a lot of health issues permanently from your life. Reversal and successful management of some of the life-long metabolic disorders can take place with the help of this intermittent fasting routine.

This routine also helps in kickstarting ketosis in your body that leads to faster fat burning. If you have oodles of fat that you want to get rid of, then this intermittent fasting routine can help in getting rid of it comparatively faster than other routines.

## Alternate Day Fasting or Eating Every Other Day

As the name is self-explanatory, this intermittent fasting requires you to remain in the fasted state for a complete 24 hours and then eat normally for the next 24 hours. There will be equal fasting and feasting windows. This is a great routine if you want to get the full benefits of intermittent fasting and yet don't want to feel left out. This routine allows you to enjoy food healthily on your eating days, and put your body in the fasting mode the other day. It gives you the best of both the worlds. Fasting for a complete 24 hours helps your body in developing the required sensitivities, and your blood sugar management also improves.

You can begin with fasting on two non-consecutive days of the week, and then add another day once you become comfortable with the routine. The major difference between this routine and One Meal a Day program is that, you would be fasting only one hour more, but would be getting a complete day for eating normally.

One Meal a Day routine makes leading a normal social life difficult as your eating window is very limited, and you can't eat unhealthy things in that window. You would be required to eat nutrient-dense food as any other meal would be unsustainable for the next 23 hours on a regular basis.

However, both routines have their own health benefits and challenges.

# Chapter 8: The Easy Way Towards 16/8 Intermittent Fasting

I have always believed that the '**easy and sustainable way**' is the **best way** as far as weight loss is concerned.

Not able to lose weight is a **BIG** problem people face all over the world. It disappoints and frustrates them. However, the **BIGGER** problem is that people are not able to maintain whatever weight they lose after they put all the effort and sacrifice. It is even more frustrating, disappointing, and heartbreaking. More than anything else, it fills them with a **Guilty Conscious** that the mistake is on their part. They are not disillusioned by the weight loss measure, but lose confidence over their ability to work consistently over anything. A few more tries, and then they stop giving it a try. That's why sustainability is more important than speed in any weight loss process.

In the beginning, when people begin their weight loss journey, they are full of zeal, enthusiasm, excitement, inspiration, and sometimes even anger and ridicule. These emotions work as fuel and drive them. However, like all emotions, these also start losing steam after a while. Tough and taxing routines soon start feeling like a burden.

People start having second thoughts about their decision to lose weight in the first place. They not only start questioning their intent, but also their ability. This happens even with those individuals who have been getting results, but aren't able to maintain them.

It is one thing to pick a rigorous routine and completely another one to keep following it in this fast-paced life full of competition and responsibilities.

People make resolutions to lose weight within a quarter, and then leave even before they have given a quarter of that time to weight loss. Thinking that one can manage any kind of routine and actually managing it with complex professional and personal life is entirely different. This happens day in and day out in the weight loss industry. Losing weight is difficult and requires great dedication and sacrifice, and that's why the success rate of the weight loss industry is so low.

This is what makes it very important why the weight loss measure should be **Highly Sustainable in the Long-Term,** and that won't happen if it isn't easy to follow.

This is where intermittent fasting; especially 16/8 intermittent fasting, emerges as a clear winner. This intermittent fasting routine is very easy to follow and requires the least effort on your part. It can be made a part of the lifestyle, and hence maintaining it would become effortless.

However, it is important that you always follow a step-by-step approach when taking up intermittent fasting.

For the successful incorporation of intermittent fasting as a way of life, it is important that you give due time to the process. You should give time to your body to adjust to the change, and must never rush the process.

# Few Important Things

## *It Is No Fad Diet*

Intermittent fasting is not a fad diet. It is a way of life our ancestors had been practicing for thousands of years. Some of the strongest animals in the world still live on the same lines. Intermittent fasting is not a technique created by some weight loss guru. It has scientific backing, and has been a part of religious, cultural, and evolutionary history. Modern intermittent fasting techniques have only done some modifications in the eating and fasting patterns for better results. More than a weight loss technique, it is a holistic way of living.

## *It Is No Magic Trick*

People are so fed up with the failure of weight loss measures, and are in such a hurry to lose weight that they start looking for magical ways to lose weight. If you also fall in this category, then you are up for disappointment. There is no magical way to lose weight. All those commercials promising weight loss through some battery powered belts, pills, powders or superfoods have been deceiving you. It takes a lot of effort and hard work on your part. You can't expect a machine to work for you and get the results. Even the people who take the help of surgeries to get rid of their weight see a weight relapse if they don't put the effort in losing and maintaining the weight.

## *It Will Take Time*

The weight doesn't come overnight, and it would definitely not go that fast. You may have to work for weeks if not months to see some result. However, the progress after you have got the first results would be fast. Thereafter, the body really gets into the fat burning mode, and hence, the results are fast, but it really takes some time to get there. If you are thinking of getting quick results, you might feel disappointed. Hence, when you get on your weight loss journey, stick to it, and remain patient.

The Results May Be Slow, but They Will Be Sustainable

The best thing about intermittent fasting is that the results may be slow to show up, but they remain sustainable. Once you start losing weight, you will be able to maintain the lost weight easily. The cases of weight relapse can only happen if you turn to the old ways of life, i.e., erratic eating. Intermittent fasting gives sustainable results, because it first helps in improving the vitals in your body that are causing weight gain. Once the vital processes improve, it starts working on burning the stored fat in the body. This step by step resolution of the problem ensures sustainability.

## *You May Need a Measuring Tape Along With the Weighing Scale to Map Your Progress*

This has been discussed even earlier in the book. It is one of the best things about intermittent fasting routine. Most weight loss routines excessively focus on calorie restriction, and that will cause nutrient deficiency. Feeling of weakness and lethargy are common and logical, as your body stops getting the required nutrition. When you lower your calorie intake, you are not only devoiding your body of extra calories, but also of nutrients, and that causes a lot of health problems. Intermittent fasting, on the other hand, doesn't restrict your calorie intake. You can take all the required nutrition from healthy food sources. It only puts a cap on the number of meals in which you can have this nutrition, and the time within which you can have it.

You would lose a considerable amount of weight in the initial phase as it happens with most weight loss measures. However, this weight loss is temporary as it is induced by a loss of water weight. Your body starts dumping excess water from the body to manage the energy deficit. However, once your body gets used to intermittent fasting, it will start burning fat in your body as fuel. This will result in loss of fat around your abdomen, thighs, and hips. However, although the fat is voluminous, it doesn't weigh much. Therefore, you may not see a significant improvement on the weighing scale as other weight loss measures promise you. But there is another side of the story too.

Intermittent fasting is a technique through which your body gets into the process of conserving and building the muscles. Most weight loss measures which boast of weight loss cannot promise prevention of muscle mass. The process of breaking and building muscles also speeds up in them. However, it is very different in intermittent fasting. It boosts the production of certain hormones in your body like the Human Growth Hormone (HGH), which helps in fat burning, while preventing the loss of muscle mass. In fact, if you follow a healthy exercise routine along with intermittent fasting, you will be able to bulk muscles faster than any other method.

Also, the feeling of weakness, lethargy, irritation, the uncontrolled and unexplained temptation for food, and other metabolic disorders don't arise in the case of intermittent fasting. After you get acclimatized, which takes only a couple of days, you start experiencing greater energy, enthusiasm, and spirit. Problems like lethargy, food cravings, and food-related irritation go away.

## Health Checkups Will Be the Best Reflectors of Your Progress

Apart from weight loss and fat burning, intermittent fasting is a way to achieve holistic health benefits. It helps in improving the overall functioning of your body. Your body is better able to cope with hypertension, heart disorders, liver problems, blood sugar control, cholesterol, oxidative stress, and chronic inflammations. Although these things will not be visible to you from the naked eye, blood tests can reflect your progress in these areas. If you want to monitor your progress, you can take blood tests at regular intervals.

## Three-Stage Process for 16/8 Intermittent Fasting Protocol

1. Elimination of Snacks
2. Shorter 12/12 fasting
3. 16/8 intermittent fasting

If you follow the procedure in the same order, you will face the least difficulty and discomfort. Your body will get the time to adjust to the change, and there would be no long-term side effects.

## Elimination of Snacks

Frequent snacking is more of a habitual issue rather than a physiological one. Most of us have become a part of modern food culture. There is food all around us. We have easy and affordable access to ready-made food that is tempting and tasty. From street food to fast food chains, the options are unlimited. Even the audio-visual mediums like television, movies, theaters, and clubs highly promote the consumption of food. This makes eating frequently a habit. Most of the times we are not eating, because we are hungry, but because the food is lying in front of us. You are never really hungry for the pop-corns while you are watching a movie. You have been actually initiated into feeling that hunger. However, that has become a part of our life, and this is among the first things that you will need to change.

You cannot have snacks. You will have to learn to transition from one meal to another without having snacks. It may sound extremely difficult, but it isn't. Slight adjustments in the composition of your meals, and a little bit of self-control will be more than enough to do the trick for you. If you still feel the urge to have something, you can have some of the permitted beverages like unsweetened fresh lime water, black tea, and coffee.

The first step towards successful implementation of intermittent fasting strategy is to eliminate all kinds of snacks from your life. You can have three meals a day. These three meals should be balanced and nutritious. You can include the food items of your choice, and you must try to remove sweets and refined carbs from these meals. Sugar-rich food items, refined carbs, aerated beverages add a lot of empty calories to your body that spikes your blood sugar levels. However, they do not give anything substantial to your gut for processing. This confuses your body as the gut begins the digestion process, but gets nothing to process. The body uses up the glucose fuel in a short while, hence, you again start feeling the hunger pangs.

Having a balanced diet that has lots of healthy fats, proteins, and fiber gives your gut the things to process. Fiber takes up a lot of space in the gut, and gets processed really slow. The same happens with fat and protein. This means that your gut would remain busy for long, and hence you wouldn't feel the hunger pangs.

69

Having a healthy diet is a good way to get rid of the habit of frequent snacking. You must also place your meals at equal intervals as that will help in creating healthy gaps between the meals.

## 12/12 Fasts

This is the easiest fasting routine to follow. You would simply need to remain in the fasted state for 12 hours, and use the remaining 12 hours for having your meals. You must use the 12 hours of your eating window to place the three meals equidistantly. Once you have gained reasonable control over your habit of snacking, it would become very easy.

Normally, we spend 7-8 hours sleeping. This is the time when you wouldn't have an urge to eat. You can have your last meal of the day 3-4 hours before bedtime, and that would do the trick. A healthy meal takes much longer than that to get processed, and hence, you wouldn't feel hunger pangs before sleeping. We generally don't have our meals as soon as we get up, and that gives us another 2-3 hour before our first meal. This means that it will be very easy to manage 12 hours of fasting in a normal routine.

The purpose of this routine is to get out of the habit of indiscriminate eating simply. This may look like overemphasizing on a simple point, but it isn't. People who have erratic sleeping patterns have a habit of eating late at night. If they don't take proper meals at night, grabbing a can of soda or munching on a pack of chips while watching TV is very common, and that can do all the damage. It will keep spiking your blood sugar levels, and the insulin resistance would keep increasing.

To remain healthy and free from insulin resistance, it is important that you strictly follow the 12-hour fasting window. You must follow this routine for a considerable period of time before moving on to the next step. It is very important that your body gets adjusted and comfortable to this schedule before you move on to the next step.

## The 16/8 Intermittent Fasting Routine

This is the real deal that you have to focus on. The 16/8 intermittent fasting routine is very easy to follow once you have got rid of the habit of snacking, and have developed the restraint to remain in the fasted state for 12 hours straight.

In this routine, you will need to remain in the fasted state for 16 hours, and will get an 8-hour eating window. It is always best to begin your fasting window early in the evening and extend it as far as possible until the next day.

If you are a morning person and wake up early, you would start feeling the urge to eat soon. Therefore, it is important that you begin your fast early in the evening. If you generally wake up between 6-7 in the morning, and like to have your breakfast between 8-9, your fasting window should begin around 5 in the evening.

If you are a night person and remain awake till late, you can have the last meal of the day a bit late and extend your first meal further into the day. However, you must try to have your last meal of the day at least 3-4 hours before going to bed. This would give your body ample time to begin the digestion process. Going to bed immediately after having your meal is never a good idea. The food never gets processed properly, and you will have digestion issues. Therefore, from a health point of view, it is important to have dinner at least 3-4 hours before hitting the bed. This also gives you the advantage that you wouldn't have to remain hungry for long once you wake up.

Remember that the urge to eat would be the strongest in the morning, and hence having dinner early in the evening helps in avoiding any kind of discomfort caused by the hunger pangs. You would be able to have food early in the day.

## Things You Will Need to Manage

### *Poor Satiety Levels*

Although I may be using the word 'easy' very liberally, to a beginner, it wouldn't be very easy. Remaining hungry is never such an easy task, especially if you are already obese. I don't say this with sarcasm, but with the knowledge that obesity can lead to hormonal imbalances that will create issues with the satiety levels of the person suffering from it.

Obese people generally also suffer from chronic inflammations in fat cells. It leads to an imbalance in the release of 'leptin' the satiety hormone. This means that you may not feel satisfied even after eating the required amount of food. You may even start feeling hunger pangs in a short while after having the meals. This happens due to leptin resistance in your body. However, this is a phenomenon that can improve once you start showing restraint on your eating habits. It may be difficult for a few days initially. However, your satiety levels would improve tremendously over a period of time.

## Food Cravings

Food cravings remain a problem in the initial days for people who have too much sugar in their diet, or eat a carbohydrate-rich diet. Sugar and refined carbs in the food lead to cravings. Simply eating something sweet doesn't solve the problem, as the more you treat yourself with sugar, the greater the urge to have it.

The best way to handle food cravings is to make some positive changes in the diet. A diet rich in fat, protein, whole grains, and fiber will not only help you in feeling a greater level of satiety, but will also eliminate the problem of frequent food cravings.

## Headaches

A nagging headache can be a problem for people starting intermittent fasting, or making a change in their diet. Once you start having a high-fat low-carb diet and lower the consumption of sugar and refined carbs, your body starts struggling to find the sugar. You will have sugar withdrawal symptoms, and the headache is one among those symptoms. The good thing is that, if you start getting the headaches, it means your body has started the transition. It indicates that you are on the right path, and your body will start experiencing fat burning soon.

To manage the headaches, you can simply take the help of unsweetened black tea or coffee. These beverages help in dealing with these headaches that may trouble you in the beginning..

## Lightheadedness

This is another problem that almost everyone faces when beginning intermittent fasting.

You can feel:

a. Your legs shaky while walking
b. Momentary darkness before your eyes when you stand up from a squatting position
c. Difficulty in maintaining balance when you stand up very quickly
d. Difficulty in concentration
e. Problems in focusing on any particular thing

All these are symptoms of sugar withdrawal, and they are **Temporary**. These symptoms will go away within a couple of days. These things happen because your body craves for sugar supply. It stops getting glucose from food at regular intervals, and it creates these symptoms as a part of its protest. However, within a few days, the body switches to burning fat for fuel, and because it is a more reliable, long-lasting, and cleaner medium of energy that even creates lower waste and toxins, these symptoms go away.

## Thoughts of Ditching the Routine

Our body has a very sophisticated fight or flight response for everything. Whenever we get into any sort of crisis, the mind creates the fight or flight response in which it tries to find the easiest way to get out of the problem. Fighting hunger is never a lucrative idea for your brain, as it may create an energy crisis. It would try to lure you into ditching the routine. It happens with every weight loss regimen. You would feel more tempted to eat things that you didn't even like in particular. Your mind would keep thinking about food all the time. You may start feeling tired, weak, and depressed. These are all feelings created to motivate you towards ditching the routine. If you want to lose weight and lead a healthy life, you will have to face them bravely and strongly for a few days as they pass away very soon.

# Chapter 9: How Intermittent Fasting Helps in Burning Fat and Losing weight?

## Modern Day Lifestyle is Greatly Responsible for the Problem

As I have already explained, the body doesn't consider fat to be a liability. On the contrary, fat is an asset to your body. It is kept for the rainy days. However, the problem begins when this fat storage reaches a threshold, and the body is not able to judge the situation wisely.

For such a complex yet sophisticated machine like the human body to make this mistake, a lot of things need to go wrong simultaneously. However, as Murphy's law states, 'Anything that can go wrong will go wrong' if you are not always guarding it ferociously.

The modern-day fast-paced life is hectic, frantic, apathetic, and competitive. Things are always running at such a pace that it is very easy to lose track of important things like health, balance in life, joy, and happiness. This is where things start to go wrong.

There was a time when food was a luxury. Our ancestors had to do all the hard work in life just to get food to the mouth. They gave great importance to food. Most rituals were woven around food.

There were rules for having food. They paid great attention to food. However, all that has changed. Today, you can get food by simply pushing a few keys on your computer, or by making a call. We are not simply working on getting food to the table. Our priorities have changed. We are now working for luxuries, and there is no limit to that.

This all leads to erratic eating habits, poor lifestyle, and high stress in life. This is where your body starts going out of balance and starts hoarding fat.

Intermittent fasting helps in creating a reasonable balance in this system. It enables your body to develop ways to cope up with the issues.

## The Process of Storing Fat

As told earlier, the body treats fat as an energy reserve. Therefore, it has a great inclination to store fat. In fact, women have a greater affinity to store fat as their body always tries to store fat for better chances of giving birth to a child. Their body fat ratio will always be greater than men. While an average male body fat ratio should be anywhere between 11-15%, the average body fat ratio in females is as high as 22-25%.

Therefore, you would always find it a struggle to keep the excess fat off your body. However, in the natural process, the energy expenditure of the body is generally the same as its energy consumption, and hence, no excess storage takes place. Some people have an overworking metabolism, and they are able to burn a lot more calories than others, hence, keeping fat off their bodies is easy for them. However, that should be treated as an exception and not as a standard case.

Whenever you eat anything, it gets broken down to calories. There are some things that are easy to break, and they supply a lot of calories easily, while others are slow and take a lot of time. However, everything you eat gets converted to calories. This is dumped into your bloodstream as glucose, and raises the blood sugar level in your body.

## Glucose as Direct Source of Energy to Cells

First of all, the glucose is used for providing energy to the cells in your body. The insulin in your body helps the cells in this process. It enables the absorption of glucose by the cells.

The energy stored in the cells will only last for a few hours. The cells need a regular supply of energy after short intervals.

## Glycogen as Energy Reserve in the Liver and Muscles

Second, the remaining glucose if left, would need to be stored quickly, as the longer the blood sugar levels remain high, the greater damage it can cause for your body. The insulin hormone then starts storing the glucose in the liver and muscles as glycogen. The glycogen stored in muscles can be used by them in case of energy storage. However, the storage is limited, and the muscles can't share this energy with other muscles. However, the energy stored in the liver as glycogen can be used for providing energy to the body in case of the energy crisis.

The energy stored in the liver as glycogen can last about 24 hours. It means once your glycogen stores are full, they can provide energy to your body for about 24 hours from the time of your last meal. However, this can only be done by the liver as the energy stored in muscles can only be used when the muscle in question needs to do some work. It can't be shared.

## Fat as Energy Reserve in the Fat Cells

Thirdly, in case there is an energy surplus; even after storing in the liver and muscles, the insulin triggers the adipose tissues or the fat cells to store the remaining energy in the form of fat. There are several layers of fat in the body. The tummy tires or oodles of fat on the belly and hips are subcutaneous fat. This is a simple energy store, and doesn't have severe health implications. The most harmful fat is the visceral fat that is deep inside the body. It starts accumulating around the vital organs and limits their ability to function properly. Chronic inflammation in this fat will also lead to several complications. More visceral fat would also mean that the oxidative stress in your body would be high. It releases a lot of free fatty acids that increase oxidative stress, and cause chronic inflammations.

However, fat of any type can be used for providing energy once your body gets in the fat burning mode. Fat in the body of an average person can provide the fuel to run the body for more than one and a half month. In fact, the fat in the body is more than sufficient to run the body for much longer than that, but other nutrient deficiencies will bring a person down.

Anyway, the fat in your body is a large energy deposit that can power your body for much longer than other energy sources. You simply need to learn the ways to use it when there is surplus fat deposit in the body.

# First Things First — The Fat Burning Mechanism

It is very important that you clearly understand the fat burning mechanism, as the lack of this knowledge keeps people confused.

Once you stop consuming food, the cells are the first to observe the energy crunch. Cells can only store a few hours worth of energy. This signals the liver to begin the process of breaking the glycogen stores. The liver metabolizes the glycogen and releases energy. This would be sufficient to run your body for 24 hours.

However, after that, your body would need more energy. In case you are not getting any supply from outside, your body would start metabolizing the fat in the body.

This is the simple math we all understand. Therefore, if you follow a restrictive calorie routine in which you lower your calorie intake below your calorie expenditure, your body will not have any other option than to burn fat.

The calculation is not that simple.

Once you lower your calorie intake, the body senses the deficit, and lowers the metabolic rate to conserve energy. It is a simple thing any prudent person would do.

God forbid, if you lose your job, you try to cut your expenses so that your savings can last much longer. No one tries to jump the gun and starts splurging, so that the reserves can be emptied faster. That's a losing strategy. You must not expect your body to be unwise.

This means that if you reduce your calorie intake by 500 calories, your body would also try to lower the calorie intake by the same amount. This adjustment helps in running the body length on the reserve fuel. It doesn't facilitate the burning of the reserve fuel.

## Why Not?

It is a very reasonable thing to ask why the body doesn't start burning the reserve fuel. There are two things in the way:

1. Your body is sensing that the energy supply hasn't cut-off; it has simply reduced. Making adjustments is a better option than splurging.
2. There is insulin floating in the blood, which will not allow metabolization of the fat cells to energy.

You need to understand that insulin is a fat storage hormone. As long as insulin is present in your blood in high quantities, it will not let the body burn fat.

Most diets ask you to lower your calorie intake, and for that, they go to extra length to explain the things to eat and the ones not to eat. Their focus is always on reducing calorie intake. So, you are allowed to have several smaller meals so that you keep feeling satiety, but never over eat calories.

This is the point where the calculations go wrong.

Every time you consume a meal, it leads to the conversion of the food into glucose and spikes the insulin levels in your blood. It takes around 8-12 hours from your last meal for the insulin levels to go down. However, if you are taking meals at regular intervals, you will not allow your body the chance to begin the process of burning fat.

You would start feeling energy drained, weak, lethargic, shaky, irritable, frustrated, and extremely tempted to eat the desired food, but would not be burning fat.

The only piece missing in this puzzle is the right condition for the initiation of fat metabolization process.

# How Does Fat Metabolization Take Place in Intermittent Fasting?

The major difference between intermittent fasting and diets is that intermittent fasting is able to create complete energy cut-off for short intervals.

## There Are 2 Important Things to Understand

**Energy Deficit**- This is a situation created by diets. The calorie intake simply goes down, but never completely stops. You still keep consuming meals at short intervals. The insulin levels in your blood still remain high due to frequent intake of food.

**Energy Cut-off** – This happens when you go into a fasting state for a considerable period of time. Here, the period of fasting is around 16 hours. However, this also means that your body gets the time once in a day when the insulin levels are really low. Remember, the insulin levels automatically dissipate after 8-12 hours.

## This Means 2 Important Things

**Favorable Condition for Burning Fat:** There are two big obstructions in the way of burning fat, and those are 1. High insulin levels, 2. Presence of high blood sugar. When you observe a fasting period of 16 hours or more, both these conditions are met. The insulin levels go down after 8-12 hours, and the blood sugar levels would be naturally low, as you wouldn't have eaten anything since long.

**Better Condition for Developing Insulin Sensitivity:** The biggest cause of insulin resistance is the over exposure of cells to the insulin hormone. However, when you start observing fasting on a regular basis, it creates a regular period of insulin absence. This makes the cells more responsive to insulin signals. It means that your cells would start responding better to insulin signals, and your pancreas will not have to pump more and more insulin into your blood.

Your body doesn't consider the complete cut off of energy supply as a deficit, but treats it as a shortage. The cells need a regular energy supply, and hence, other modes of energy supply are engaged. The glycogen stores get metabolized first. However, they are small, and when the body starts drawing energy from the glycogen stores regularly, they don't last long. It means that soon, the glycogen stores would get empty, and they would not get restored on a daily basis during the eating windows. Therefore, during the fasting window, your body will have to start burning the fat for providing energy to the cells.

The energy provided by your last meal wouldn't last very long. The body would start looking for more energy. Your glycogen stores would be weak as you would be drawing energy from them. Within a few hours, your body would have no other option than to begin the metabolization of fat for energy.

Here, it is important to remember that by the time your body reaches this stage, around 6-8 hours would have passed. Intermittent fasting improves the insulin sensitivity of your body, and hence, the insulin present in your body would already be low. This would create an ideal situation for fat metabolization.

## The Magical Phase of Ketosis

Ketosis is a phenomenon in which our body starts burning fat as fuel. This process can solve all your worries about burning fat.

Let us understand the process clearly:

Our body can survive on 2 types of fuel:

1. Glucose
2. Fat

### Glucose

We get glucose fuel through a carbohydrate-rich diet. Our body breaks the carbs into glucose and uses it as a fuel. Glucose is an easy to use fuel, and our body loves it. Most cells can directly use glucose as the main fuel. However, the problem with glucose is that it doesn't last long. It also keeps raising your blood sugar levels, causing an insulin spike.

### Fat

Fat is another form of fuel our body can use. Our body can use nutritional fat as well as the body fat for producing cleaner energy that lasts long. The process to use fat as energy is known as ketosis. It is the alternative source of energy that your body can use.

Historically, ketosis had been the original way of producing energy. Humankind started as a hunter-gatherer. Even the idea of a carb-rich diet didn't exist back them. Our ancestors lived entirely on animal fat and protein obtained from the hunt and whatever carb came into the system was from gathering fruits and shoots. However, herbs, shrubs, fruits, and shoots were never a favorite medium of food.

Fat and protein made up most of the diet, and hence, ketosis was the only way our body was running. We can again make that happen by bringing some changes in our diet and intermittent fasting.

Ketosis is a healthy way to live, and it helps in losing weight very fast. Your body always remains in the fat burning mode, and hence, as soon as the fat from nutrition ends, the body starts burning the body fat. It doesn't have to make any transition at all. This is the reason ketogenic diet, which is high-fat, high-protein and low-carb diet has become so much popular for losing weight these days.

A ketogenic diet alone can help in losing a considerable amount of fat quickly. If you follow a ketogenic diet along with intermittent fasting, the benefits will get multiplied, and you would be able to lose weight much faster.

The problem with fat burning through any other process is that it would require making a transition from burning glucose fuel to fat fuel, and the body take a lot of time in making the switch. If you feel that you can force your body to make this switch twice a day, the process won't remain efficient and effective.

That's why if you want to lose weight quickly through intermittent fasting, you will need to make corrective changes to your diet.

## Help from Fat Burning Hormones

When your body is in a fasting state while you are asleep, it also increases the production of HGH. This hormone also facilitates faster burning of fat and building of muscles.

In this way, intermittent fasting creates an ideal situation for improving your health as well as burning fat for energy.

The 16 hours gap between the meals gives your body ample time to target the fat stores. The absence of insulin means that there would be no roadblocks in the metabolization of the fat stores. Therefore, the body starts the process of burning fat.

## Advantages of High-Intensity Interval Training (HIIT) in the Fasted State

When you do HIIT in the fasted state, you raise your energy demands greatly. However, your body is still in the fasted state, and it isn't getting energy supply from outside. It means it will have any other option than to burn fat for producing the required energy.

The longer you work out, the more fat your body will be able to burn.

This is the reason why all the experts advise doing exercise in the fasted state as it helps in burning fat. You can speed up your fat burning process by doing HIIT on alternate days, and by doing normal exercises on the other days of the week. HIIT also helps in the building of specific muscles in the body. The production of HGH is also high in the body during the fasted state, and that also helps in faster fat burning and muscle building. It also increases your endurance, and hence, you will be able to exercise for longer periods without facing many difficulties.

The muscles in the body have their own glycogen stores, and doing HIIT in the fasted state enables them to utilize their glycogen stores, hence, you don't really feel muscle fatigue to a great extent.

In the following chapters, we will discuss the ways in which men and women can follow intermittent fasting for faster fat burning, and other health benefits. Although most things remain the same in case of fasting for men and women, there are some fine things that are different, hence, need to be kept in mind.

Therefore, we will discuss 16/8 intermittent fasting for men and women separately.

# Chapter 10: 16/8 Intermittent Fasting for Men

The 16/8 intermittent fasting protocol for men is among the most successful and widely followed ways to lose weight and gain good health.

You can divide your day into 2 parts:

- The Fasting Window
- The Eating Window

The best thing about 16/8 intermittent fasting is that it can be made a part of your daily life. It doesn't ask you to do anything extra, and hence, it is easy to follow. There are only two things to be kept in mind.

1. The hours within which you can eat
2. The things you should eat

The success of any weight loss plan depends on your dedication to that plan, and intermittent fasting is no exception. Although intermittent fasting puts no holds on the things you can eat and the things you can't. Yet, it is expected of you to show a reasonable attitude towards food items.

- ✓ You **shouldn't** eat unhealthy things
- ✓ You **can't** eat things in excess quantities
- ✓ You **mustn't** eat outside your eating window

# The Fasting Window

The fasting window should generally begin early in the evening, when you are about to finish the active part of the day. There are several benefits to beginning the fasting window at the end of the day.

❖ You'd get in the resting mode

❖ Your chances of getting invited to eat something by friends and colleagues would get low

❖ You'd be at a more relaxed atmosphere

❖ Your body would get at least 3-4 hours to digest the food before you hit the bed. Your gut would be really grateful for that.

Ideally, the fasting window should begin anywhere between 5-7 in the evening. Men should fast for at least 16 hours,  which means if you begin your fast around 5 in the evening, you will be able to have the first meal of the day around 9.

If you take it at 7 in the evening, the first meal would not be possible before 11 in the day.

Pushing it any further can keep pushing the first meal of the day farther into the day.

This may not look like a big issue at the moment, but believe me; it's something you should worry about. It takes around 4-5 hours before your gut is able to properly process a healthy meal; therefore, it is very unlikely that you would feel any hunger pang before hitting the bed. However, things would be different when you wake up.

Even if you sleep for 7-8 hours, the total fasting time would have been around 12 hours when you wake up. This is the time the hunger starts to build up. If you maintain a healthy exercise routine, you wouldn't feel very hungry for another 1-2 hours as physical activity suppresses the feeling of hunger momentarily. However, the hunger would start building up pretty strongly after that.

I am assuming that you would also need to go to work. Passing the next one or two hours in the fasted state while working can be difficult. Therefore, it is always best to begin the fasting window early, so that you can get the first meal of the day before you start the active part of the day.

- ✓ Begin your fasting window as early as possible, and try to make it a routine.
- ✓ Don't shift the timings a lot as your body would also need to adjust to the routine
- ✓ It is important that you somewhat fix the timings of your first and last meal of the day

# Eating Window

You get 8 hours for the eating window. These 8 hours are important as you will need to take all the nutrition during these 8 hours. It may look like a lot of time, but it isn't. After 16 hours of fasting, when you have the first meal of the day, it is generally very difficult to have another meal after an interval of 4 hours.

You will also need to ensure that you don't indulge in overeating.

If you don't have a properly balanced meal, transitioning from one meal to another smoothly without the urge to have something in between will become difficult.

Therefore, it is important that you have a very balanced first meal of the day.

It should have all the macronutrients, and should provide the required minerals and vitamins that your body needs.

The first meal of the day is important as it is going to be the most fulfilling meal for you. It is always best that you get it at home. You get complete control over the ingredients of your meal, and the way you prepare it. If you have your meals out, you can't be sure of these things.

You must always remember that food is a very important part of any weight loss strategy, therefore, you can't ignore this part completely.

Although you can have 3 meals in the 8 hours eating window, it is generally not possible to have 3 proper meals in this short gap. If you have a healthy and fulfilling meal at the start of the day, you are not likely to have the urge to have a complete meal at lunch.

The lunch should be light as it can make you feel lethargic. Generally, the last meal of the day is the second proper meal you will be able to have, and that's why you will have to focus on the first and last meal.

# Exercise

Exercise is another important part of an intermittent fasting routine. Intermittent fasting helps your body in getting into the fat burning mode. However, it is your job to create the energy demand. If you are leading a highly active life, then that can come naturally, but the chances of the same are slim. This makes it important that you create the energy demands through exercise.

High-Intensity Interval Training is one of the best ways to create high energy demands quickly. It pushes your body to burn calories faster. Intermittent fasting also leads to an increase in the production of HGH in your body, and that also helps in increasing your fat burning abilities through exercise.

✓ You will need to remain in the fasted state for at least 16 hours in a day to get the maximum benefits.
✓ The longer you would fast, the better the results would be.

- ✓ You should try to extend the fasting hours as much as possible.
- ✓ The best strategy to do so would be to begin the fasting early, and start pushing the breakfast later into the day.
- ✓ You should reduce the intake of refined carbs and sugar in your diet.
- ✓ You should also reduce your reliance on processed food items as much as possible.
- ✓ The shift towards the whole and unprocessed food items.
- ✓ Drink plenty of fluids.
- ✓ You can have unsweetened black tea and coffee, and even fresh lime water for suppressing the hunger pangs.
- ✓ However, you should avoid excessive consumption of tea or coffee in both the fasting as well as eating windows.
- ✓ You must take as much rest as possible.
- ✓ Sleeping for at least 7-8 hours is very important for faster weight loss.

# Chapter 11: 14/10 Intermittent Fasting for Women

Although the basic idea of intermittent fasting remains the same for both men and women, some important differences need to be kept in mind.

The body of a woman is highly sensitive to hunger. Fasting for extended periods without proper preparation can throw the hormonal balance of a woman's body off balance.

Women should fast for fewer hours, and should have a longer eating window. Studies have shown that fasting for 14 hours and having a 10-hour eating window yields better weight loss results for women.

## Reason for Shorter Fasting Window

The body of a woman is more sensitive to hunger signals. The food not only provides energy to the physical body, but it also provides psychological security. Once it reaches puberty till it reaches menopause, a woman's body is designed always to remain ready to bear a child. Bringing a new life into this world is a big responsibility, and the body of a woman understands this. That's why women naturally have a greater body fat ratio. They have stronger cravings for food, and weaker tolerance to hunger pangs.

Several studies show that psychological insecurities are also associated with hunger. This is one reason why women are more prone to emotional eating than men.

Beginning longer fasting routines without putting your body into the habit can disturb the delicate hormonal balance in a woman's body. It can also affect the fertility and ability to produce children. A woman may experience lower libido if she starts longer fasting routines without acclimatizing her body.

Therefore, it is important that women should always start with shorter routines and then move on to longer fasts. Although they can follow longer fasting protocols for some time once they get used to it, the best and sustainable results come when they follow shorter fasting routines like 14/10. In any case, women shouldn't fast longer than 24 hours. It can be really hard on their bodies, and can cause serious hormonal imbalance.

# Ways to Achieve Better Weight Loss Results

## Healthy Diet

A healthy diet is very helpful as far as weight loss is considered. Although achieving weight loss simply through diet is difficult in practice, but when you use it with intermittent fasting, the results can be outstanding.

Here, it is important that diet here doesn't imply calorie restriction. The meaning of diet is a combination of all the macronutrients in a healthy proportion and consumption of all the required minerals and vitamins.

A woman's body reacts differently to food than a man's body. Men may not gain that much weight or fat from the same food, whereas it can be a completely different story for women. Therefore, women should choose the components of food wisely.

- ✓ Eating as much whole food as possible is always the best.
- ✓ Avoiding processed and refined foods will help a lot in losing weight faster.
- ✓ Women should completely avoid sugar, and refined carb-rich food items as these lead to excessive food cravings.
- ✓ They should also avoid soda and other sweetened beverages.
- ✓ Focus on fresh foods and green leafy vegetables.
- ✓ They should drink plenty of fluids to remain hydrated, and it also helps in flushing out toxins

## Exercise

Exercise is a healthy way to stay fit and lose weight. Irrespective of gender, exercise has a positive impact on overall health. As far as women are concerned, they can get great help in losing weight through exercise. It not only helps in burning calories, but also proves to be a great stress buster.

- ➢ Women should try to achieve a balance between High-intensity exercises and light exercises.
- ➢ Walking, jogging, swimming, yoga, and aerobic exercises along with heavy exercises can help them in remaining fit.

## Active Lifestyle

Maintaining an active lifestyle is more important for a healthy body. A woman's body is more prone to weight gain. Therefore, maintaining an active lifestyle helps them better in remaining in shape.

# Chapter 12: Nutrition

Intermittent fasting is very lenient as far as nutrition is concerned. By being lenient means, you are not restricted from eating anything in particular. You can eat pretty much anything within reasonable limits once in a while. It means if you have to attend a birthday party of a friend or any other celebration, then you wouldn't have to think a million times before having a piece of cake, or any other dessert.

You can enjoy a piece without carrying the burden of guilt upon yourself. However, this liberty comes with a caveat. You must eat it within reasonable limits. This liberty helps in keeping the temptations away. People who are tied under restrictions in eating often feel depressed and crushed. It leads to pessimism and negativity.

Remember, intermittent fasting is less about what you eat, and more about when you eat. As long as you are following the fasting hours, your body will be able to bear the once in a while indulgences.

Intermittent fasting limits the number of hours within which you can eat. It can mean a lot for people who have a habit of snacking frequently. Intermittent fasting schedule would limit the number of meals you can take, and hence, you will have to draw your whole nutrition from 2-3 meals within the 8-10 hours eating window.

Moving on from one meal to another can get difficult if you are not having balanced meals. If you are consuming too many refined carbs, then also, you might find it difficult to move on from one meal to another without feeling the food cravings and hunger pangs.

Therefore, it is very important that you have a very balanced meal.

## Managing the Macronutrients

There are 3 main components of any meal

1. Fat
2. Protein
3. Carbohydrate

You must consume all these macronutrients in a balanced manner. Having a nutrient dense meal always helps in curbing hunger pangs for long, and suppressing the food cravings.

The ideal distribution of the macronutrients should be in the ratio given below:

### Fat: 70-75%

Fat is dense, and the body takes a lot of time to process fats. This means that when you consume a fat-rich diet, it keeps you feeling full for longer, and prevents hunger pangs. The body takes much longer in processing the fats, and this also helps in preventing the insulin spike in your body. You can easily get a lot of calories even by eating fat in small quantities. When you have to consume a lot of calories in fewer meals, making fat the main component of your meal always helps.

However, you must ensure that you eat healthy fats. You can get healthy fats from animal meat, fish, nuts, seeds, and fruits. 1 gram of fat provides 9 calories. It is more than double the number of calories received from carbs of the same weight. This means you can get more calories by consuming fat in smaller quantities. You must include healthy fats in your diet to stay satiated.

## Protein: 20-25%

Protein is essential for your muscles building. When your body is running on a low-carb diet, and you are doing a lot of exercises, there is a loss of muscle mass. The muscles are constantly breaking, and new ones are building. To help this process, you will need to consume a lot of protein. Therefore, protein should form the second biggest part of your meals. However, you should never consume protein in excess as that would again get broken as glucose.

You can get protein from lean meats, fish, nuts, dairy, egg white, and legumes. Try to have protein in moderate amounts to ensure that you get the required protein from your meals.

## Carbohydrate: 5-10%

Carbohydrate should constitute the smallest part of your meal. You must not consume refined carbs as they get processed very quickly, and increase the blood sugar levels. However, once the body processes the refined carbs, you would start feeling hungry again.

Consumption of refined carbs would lead to food cravings and hunger pangs.

You must consume complex carbohydrates like whole grains that take a lot of time to get processed, and give your gut a lot of fiber in the end. This not only helps in keeping your blood sugar levels low, but is also very good for your gut ecosystem. There are several important trace minerals that are only found in whole grains, and that's why they are so important.

Green leafy vegetables are the second most important source of carbohydrates that you must consume. Green leafy vegetables do not only have a lot of fiber, but also vitamins and minerals in huge quantities. They help you with a lot of antioxidants, phytonutrients, and flavonoids that are helpful in fighting chronic inflammations. You must consume at least 7-8 cups of green leafy vegetables every day for a healthy body.

There are several benefits of consuming green leafy vegetables in large quantities. First, they are very low in calories, and hence you can consume them in any quantity you like without worrying about the calories consumed. Second, the green leafy vegetables provide a gel-like fiber to your body that helps your gut a lot. It helps in keeping your digestive system clean. You wouldn't face problems like constipation and other such issues. Third, green leafy vegetables can be consumed in large quantities, and hence they help you in feeling fuller for longer.

You can eat them as salads, or even make a smoothie as per your liking. However, it is always advisable to avoid starchy vegetables in large quantities, as they just add calories to your system and raise your blood sugar levels.

## Things to Avoid

* Fruit Juices: It is never advisable to have fruit juices. Fresh or packed, fruit juices are not good for your body. They raise your blood sugar levels instantly without adding fiber to your system. Drinking juice is like adding empty calories to your system.
* Soda and other caloric beverages: Like juices, they also add empty calories to your system. In addition, they are even worse for your body as they are prepared from refined sugar. You will start feeling cravings to have more soon after you have some.
* Refined flours: Refined flours and the products made from them are bad for your health. These flours do not have the original fiber content, and are very easy to process. This means that after consuming refined flours, you will again start feeling hungry very soon. They are bad for your digestive system and raise your blood sugar levels very fast.
* Sugar: Sugar in any form should be avoided. You must buy everything after checking the label. If it has sugar, maple syrup, fructose, or any other such thing at the top of the ingredient list, it must be avoided. Such things will make

your fasting routine very difficult as you will have food cravings and frequent hunger pangs.

❖ Processed Food: Processed food items are bad for your health. To increase the shelf life of processed food items, a lot of sugar is added to them. In place of healthy fats, trans fats and hydrogenated fats are used. All these things are very bad for your health, hence, you must avoid them at all costs.

❖ Trans Fats: Trans fats are bad, and although most processed food items don't have trans fat listed as an ingredient, or its value is given as zero, it is not the whole truth. The best way is to avoid highly processed food items, especially the ones with a lot of added preservatives

# Chapter 13: Exercise

Exercising is important as it helps in burning fat faster. It is also important for building healthier muscles. All those people who have been objecting exercise in a fasted state only explain one side of the story.

There are a few things on which everyone agrees:

1. Exercises help in burning fat
2. They help in keeping the body fit
3. They also help in uplifting your mood and bringing positivity

Now, some experts believe that when you exercise in the fasted state, your body feels the energy crunch, and tries to break muscles as calories. This will happen because, after carbs end, the muscles are the easiest form of energy. The muscles are made of protein, and protein can also be broken down easily. However, it isn't that simple.

Although it is correct that some muscle loss takes place while you are doing exercise, it is wrong to assume that it happens because your body is trying to produce energy from them. Some amount of loss of muscle mass would take place even after you have had a high dose of glucose drink. This happens because the muscles are continuously getting damaged during exercise, and they break apart to give way to stronger ones.

Once your body has exhausted the glucose and glycogen reserves, it starts burning the fat reserves for energy. The fat is a more reliable and long-lasting source of energy, and it can fulfill all the energy needs of the body without causing any harm. To think that the body would think or behave otherwise is irrational.

## The HGH Story

Our body produces an amazing hormone by the name of Human Growth Hormone. The production of this hormone is very high during our growing years as it helps in the building of bones, muscles, and every other part of our body. The production of this hormone is at its peak when we reach puberty, as we start growing at an immense rate all of a sudden. However, as soon as we cross our teens, the production of this hormone slows down as our body realizes that it has stopped growing at a fast pace.

However, our body never stops producing HGH completely. It keeps producing this hormone is short spurts. It is still a hormone that helps in growth and repair. So whenever you are in trauma or great pain, the production of this hormone increases.

Under normal circumstances, there are some specific conditions under which the production of HGH increases:

- When you are sleeping
- When the production of 'ghrelin', the hunger hormone is high in your gut

- When the insulin levels are the lowest in your gut

When you are in the fasted state, all these 3 conditions mentioned above are met. This increases the production of HGH in your body. This hormone can do some wonderful things. Among others, some important things are:

- ✓ It improves your stamina
- ✓ It accelerates fat burning
- ✓ It prevents loss of muscle mass
- ✓ It helps in the building new muscles

This means that when you do high-intensity exercise in the fasted state, the HGH in your blood would help in burning fat faster, and would also support building new muscles.

Therefore, you can exercise in the fasted state without having to worry a lot. The only thing you need to remember is that always increase your exercise timings slowly. Never start with bigger sets. Always build up your routine in stages.

# HIIT

High-Intensity Interval Training is very helpful in burning fat, as you get to create huge energy demands that are to be met by burning fat. However, you must remember that HIIT puts a lot of pressure on your body, and hence, you must give your body the due rest after exercise.

HIIT should always be carried out on alternate days, so that the body gets proper rest and recovery time. On the alternate days when you are not doing HIIT, you can do light exercises like walking, jogging, swimming, yoga, and aerobic exercises.

# Some Golden Rules to Safely Exercise While Fasting

### Do HIIT Near the End of Your Fasting Schedule

If you keep your exercise routine close to the time of your ending the fast, you can get calories very soon. This is a good way to put a stop to all doubts of muscle loss. A protein rich diet at the end of your HIIT will help in removing all fears of muscle loss. It would also provide you the required energy.

### Always Remain Hydrated

Dehydration can be more dangerous than the calorie deficit. You must always drink plenty of fluids to remain hydrated. Fasting only stops you from consuming calories. It has nothing against remaining hydrated. It is important for flushing out toxins and running the body smoothly.

### Smaller Sets for Shorter Duration

The purpose of HIIT is to create sudden energy demands. If you stretch HIIT for too long, it can cause problems like muscle cramps. You must do small sets and keep taking breaks.

## *Always Listen to Your Body*

Your fight must be against the fat and other physical ailments, but it isn't against your body. You must always listen to your body and pay heed to its demands. If you ever feel that the routine is getting overtaxing, you should take a break.

# Chapter 14: Things to Be Careful Of

## Pay Due Attention to Your Nutrition

Nutrition is very important for health. You must never forget that intermittent is not just a way to lose weight, but also a method to achieve good health. Weight loss and fat burning are simply a consequence of good health. You can't get healthy without proper nutrition. You will get a limited number of meals in a day, and you will have to take all the nutrition from those meals only. Hence, you will have to eliminate all the unnecessary things from your meals. You must choose healthy things that can provide you the required nutrition and help in your weight loss goals.

You will have to remove useless things like chips, cookies, crackers, bagels, donuts, etc. that are made up of refined carbs and sugar, which will only add empty calories to your system. You must consume a nutrient dense diet.

## Don't Show Haste

Most people are in a haste to lose weight. They forget that losing weight can be a very taxing, frustrating, and time-consuming task. Your body needs to make a switch from fat storing mode to fat burning mode. A lot of changes are required from your lifestyle to your eating patterns. If you show haste, you may start following things by the book, but you wouldn't be able to maintain them for long.

Intermittent fasting will only bring sustainable results for you if you are able to make it a part of your daily routine. Otherwise, it will be difficult to get results, and even if you do get some results, they will vanish away very soon.

## Overenthusiasm Can Be Dangerous

People are ready to make any kind of compromise to lose their weight and get good health. They would agree to sweat in the gym two hours a day, or not eating candy ever in their lives again. However, these are promises made in overenthusiasm to get results, they are never sustainable, and in fact, dangerous to a certain degree. Your body needs time to adjust to lifestyle changes. The way of life you have been following hasn't developed all of a sudden. Your body has been following it for decades. If you'd try to make a sudden switch, it would only bring poor results.

You will have to give your body the time to adjust. You must not start with any hard intermittent fasting routine. It is always best to start by eliminating snacks. Then move ahead by creating healthy gaps between meals. Once your body gets used to it, start fasting for shorter intervals like 12 hours or so. Once you have got used to it then only move to fast for 14-16 hours or longer.

Never, and I repeat never, ever begin with longer fasts to get instant results. Our body doesn't work that way. If you would try giving a jolt to your system, you may trigger adverse reactions that would become difficult to handle, and may even lead to medical emergencies.

## Limit Your Tea and Coffee Intake

Unsweetened black tea or coffee can be of great help when you begin intermittent fasting. They help in relieving the sugar withdrawal symptoms and the headache arising from it. They also help a lot in suppressing hunger. However, they shouldn't be used as a regular medium to suppress hunger.

The feeling of hunger is beneficial for your body to a great extent. It kickstarts the fat burning process. Apart from that, too much tea and coffee can be bad for your health.

## Avoid Dehydration and Overhydration

Water is important in fasting. Your body is devoid of calories, and it starts the cleaning process to optimize the bodily processes. This leads to the dumping of a lot of water. In case you stop drinking a reasonable quantity of water to stay hydrated, it can cause health issues like dehydration. It may also lead to the formation of kidney stones, as a lot of decalcification is also taking place in the body. The best way to avoid this problem is to keep drinking water at regular intervals. You must drink water whenever you feel thirsty. Never try to suppress your thirst.

As it is important to ensure that you remain hydrated, it is also important that you ensure that overhydration doesn't take place. Too much water intake can also cause problems, as it would put a lot of undue pressure on your kidneys. It is important to reach a balance.

# Don't Remain Overobsessed About Food

Fasting requires abstaining from food for a considerable period of time in a day. However, some people can abstain from food physically, but mentally, they are always thinking about food. This can have a serious psychological impact, and would also affect the weight loss process. Such an attitude would also lead to binge eating, and it always results in gaining more weight.

While in the fasting state, you must keep yourself busy, so that your mind is not always focused on food. The more occupied you are, the less likely you would think about food.

# Social and Emotional Eating Can Be Bad

If you are an emotional eater or eat under social pressure, it can become difficult for you to lose weight. It is less about consuming some extra calories, but more about showing restraint or self-control. The lower self-control you have over your eating, the difficult it would be for you to avoid piling up of calories, or cheating on regular days.

## Don't Treat Intermittent Fasting as Magic

Intermittent fasting is a way to lose weight. It is no magic trick. It is a simple, tried, and tested way of life that our ancestors had been leading for thousands of years. We have strayed from that path in the past few centuries, and that has led to the outbreak of this obesity epidemic.

Intermittent fasting only helps you in mending your ways and lifestyle. Weight loss and other health benefits come because your body gets into a better position to fight the ailments. However, if you start treating intermittent fasting as a magic trick, and stop putting in real effort to lose weight, you may never see any result. To lose weight, it is important that you remain sincere in your endeavor and be patient in your behavior.

# Chapter 15: Some Specific Health Benefits of 16/8 Intermittent Fasting

Weight loss and fat burning are some of the most talked about health benefits of 16/8 intermittent fasting routine. However, the health benefits are simply not limited to weight loss. Intermittent fasting is a way to bring holistic health benefits.

It is a way of life that helps in improving the overall health biomarkers. You not only start looking fit from outside, but get fit from inside. It is a way to improve on many physiological parameters. It will help you in managing your blood sugar levels. It will also help you in dealing with your high blood pressure. If you are suffering from chronic inflammations, you will see improvement in it. If you have been struggling with cholesterol issues, intermittent fasting can help even in that area too.

Given below are some of the most important health benefits that can bring a positive change in your life.

## Better Blood Sugar Control

Blood sugar management is directly related to insulin sensitivity. Apart from the people who are suffering from type 1 diabetes, most people face blood sugar management issues because their cells stop responding properly to the insulin signals. As a result, the blood sugar levels remain unreasonably high for longer periods; leading to several health complications.

However, insulin resistance is always at the core of this problem. If you want to have better control over your blood sugar levels, there can be no better way than intermittent fasting. It is the most reliable way to improve insulin sensitivity in your body. Your body will be able to lower the blood sugar levels faster, hence, you will be able to prevent a debilitating problem like diabetes forever. Diabetes never comes alone. It brings with itself several other health complications too. It is always best to keep this disease at bay.

Unfortunately, if you are already suffering from the problem, you must consult your physician before beginning intermittent fasting. People already suffering from diabetes would need a frequent dose adjustment of their medication, and also close monitoring of their blood sugar levels. Fasting for long can cause blood sugar levels to fluctuate at times, hence, it wouldn't be advisable to follow intermittent fasting without discussing with your doctor.

## Improved Heart Health

Every year, more than 635,000 people die of heart-related disorders in the US alone. It is the number one cause of preventable deaths here. We all know that heart problems are a leading cause of death. We also know that most of us are likely to develop issues causing heart problems. Yet, we remain blissfully ignorant. Poor lifestyle, unhealthy choice of food items, and bad eating habits along with excessive stress, are the main things that cause heart problems.

However, we don't really do anything at all about most of these things. We keep blaming high cholesterol in our food most of the times for all the heart problems. Food manufacturing companies also keep marketing cholesterol as the main problem and never really focus on the real reasons.

Dietary cholesterol doesn't even constitute 20% of the total cholesterol in our body. Most of the cholesterol in the body is produced inside our body.

The cholesterol is a building block for some of the most important hormones and also the cell structures. Without cholesterol, your heart may bleed to death. It is the main component that repairs the damage caused to your heart vessels.

Cholesterol is not the chief cause of the problems. Diabetes or high blood sugar can be the main cause, as it thickens the arteries and increases stiffness. The arteries are not able to expand when required.

High blood pressure is also a big reason for most heart problems, as it causes a lot of ischemic heart injuries. Your heart is pumping gallons of blood every day. During the course of its functioning, it keeps facing injuries. Whenever there is an injury, the cholesterol rushes to that part to mend the area which gets damaged. This repair and patchwork cause the heart vessels to thicken.

Sometimes, the patchwork ruptures and forms blood clots that also cause blockages in the heart. However, cholesterol was never the cause of the problem in the first place. High blood sugar, high blood pressure, chronic inflammations in the heart region, high oxidative stress, are among the reasons that lead to heart problems.

Intermittent fasting helps you in dealing with all of these problems at the same time:

It helps in bringing down consistent high-blood sugar levels by improving insulin sensitivity. Due to a long gap between the meals, your blood sugar levels naturally start remaining low, hence, that also eases some pressure from your heart too.

Insulin resistance also leads to a high blood pressure problem. As the insulin resistance goes down in the body with the help of intermittent fasting, so does the blood pressure issue gets solved. It eliminates another cause of heart and kidney damage.

Visceral fat is the main cause of chronic inflammations in your body. It increases the oxidative stress in the body, and releases a lot of free fatty acids that cause chronic inflammations. Intermittent fasting helps in reducing the levels of visceral fat. It also helps your body in using free fatty acids for metabolization to produce energy. This again lowers the risk of heart issues as well as chronic inflammation.

When the free fatty acids go down in your body, the oxidative stress starts decreasing automatically.

# Improved Mental Acuity

The brain is one of the most important organs in the body. It is crucial for our survival. We are called an intelligent race because of our developed brain. However, in the past few decades, there has been a significant increase in the cases of neurodegenerative disorders like Alzheimer's and Parkinson's disease. More and more people are getting affected by these problems, and the age of onset of these problems has also decreased. Meaning, people are getting affected by these issues quite early in their lives.

It is a condition that affects more than 5 million people in the US. Studies show that the risk of death due to this condition has increased by 89%. Yet, very little is done to prevent it. As per the experts, it is estimated that around 16 million people will be facing this condition by 2050.

The main cause of most neurodegenerative disorders is lower production of new cells. Like all other cells in our body, the brain cells also multiply, get old, die, and then regenerate. This keeps our brain forever, young and active. With age, people get smarter, sharper, and wiser. The process of the birth of new brain cells or neurons is called neurogenesis. For carrying out neurogenesis, a special type of protein known as Brain-Derived Neurotrophic Factor (BDNF) is required. However, oxidative stress, the presence of free radicals, and lower levels of antioxidants can lead to a decrease in the production of BDNF. It would also impact the process of neurogenesis and neuroplasticity.

These things lead to the problems, and the ability of the brain to function for long gets low. People start having problems with basic functionality of the brain like remembering things.

Intermittent fasting has emerged as a ray of hope in this direction. Several studies indicate that intermittent fasting can increase the production of BDNF considerably. This would mean that your brain would be able to function better as the production of new cells wouldn't get affected. It would lead to an improvement in mood, memory, focus, and other cognitive functions of practicing individuals.

Strokes have second place in the list. They claim more than 140,000 lives every year. The causes are a poor lifestyle, bad eating habits, stress, hypertension, diabetes,etc.

Studies show that higher production of BDNF and antioxidants can also help in preventing stroke-related deaths.

Not only this, but intermittent fasting can also help in improving the condition of people suffering from epileptic seizures. Studies have proven that one of the major reasons for these seizures is excessive dependence on sugar fuel. Intermittent fasting helps in reducing the dependence on sugar fuel. The carb intake goes down, and people with this problem show considerable improvement.

# Reduction in the Risk of Chronic Inflammations

Free radicals and oxidative stress are some of the terms you may be hearing a lot these days. The free radicals are nothing more than uncharged particles that haven't been used yet. Our body keeps producing free radicals as byproducts of various simple functions like cellular reactions, food metabolism, breathing, and other vital functions. Level free radicals don't pose any threat, and can also be used for fighting pathogens in the body or providing immunity. The antioxidants in the body maintain a balance between the free radicals, and also prevent free radical damage.

However, over time, free radical damage can increase and may lead to chronic inflammations. Free radical damage increases when your body gets too dependent on glucose fuel as it releases a lot of free radicals. The greater the free radicals in your body, the higher will be the oxidative stress, and you would become prone to chronic inflammations.

The best way to manage the problem is to follow intermittent fasting, and follow a high-fat low-carb diet. Increasing the intake of food items rich in antioxidants also helps in lowering the risk of free radical damage.

Chronic inflammations are responsible for causing most of the health issues. These are very difficult to detect as they silently keep developing inside your body without showing symptoms. They can make your vital functions ineffective. The best way to prevent chronic inflammations is to lead a healthy lifestyle, improve the intake of antioxidant-rich food items, reduce dependence on carb-rich food, and practice intermittent fasting.

## Improved Satiety

One of the biggest problems faced by people suffering from weight issues is that they are never able to feel fully satiated from food. Although they may not feel significant hunger, they can't stop eating. Most of the times, this becomes a reason for social ridicule. However, it is not a thing to be laughed at. It is a physiological disorder caused by chronic inflammation in the fat cells, and it is known as 'Leptin Resistance.'

The hippocampus of the brain has the responsibility to receive signals from your body and transmit the message to you. For instance, when your fat stores get full, the hippocampus sends you a signal that you need to stop eating. You start feeling full all of a sudden. The gut sends the hippocampus ghrelin signals, and you start feeling hungry.

The fat cells release a hormone called leptin that sends the signal of satiety whenever you are full. When you are hungry, the leptin levels are the lowest in your blood, as they start rising as you start eating. The leptin levels would be the highest after 10-20 minutes of your having a full meal. It takes a while for your brain to receive the signal that your stomach is completely full.

However, you soon start to realize that the stomach is getting full, and your eating intensity and taste starts reducing. Sadly, that stops happening when a person is suffering from leptin resistance.

This problem is caused by inflammation in the fat cells. The fat cells start releasing leptin hormones at a steady rate. This means that in place of releasing the leptin hormone only when the stomach is full, the fat cells keep releasing it at a steady rate even when you have an empty stomach. This causes overexposure of the hippocampus to the hormone signal, and it stops registering the signal and reacting to it.

This means that you will never feel fully satisfied with food ever. Even when you have eaten more than required, you may not mind eating a bit more. This problem is more problematic for obese people, as they are never able to have any calorie restriction.

Intermittent fasting can help in resolving this problem slowly. When you fast for longer periods, the intake of food is stopped for long. The fat cells still keep releasing the leptin hormone, but the intensity never increases as the provocation of food is not there. This lowers the release of the leptin hormone. Slowly and gradually, the brain again develops sensitivity to the leptin signals, and things improve.

If you also start consuming antioxidant-rich food, the situation can be improved even faster.

These are some of the common health issues faced these days, and the ways in which intermittent fasting can help in solving them.

Intermittent fasting is not only a way to lose weight and burn fat, but it is also a way to attain optimum health by improving important health biomarkers.

# Chapter 16: Who Shouldn't Practice Intermittent Fasting

Intermittent fasting is a fascinating concept with great health benefits, and lowest risk factors. But it still poses a risk for some individuals. People with high energy needs, eating disorders, and diabetes shouldn't practice intermittent fasting.

People Falling in These Groups Shouldn't Practice Intermittent Fasting

## Pregnant Women

Some experts say that pregnant mothers can practice intermittent fasting till the first trimester or can tweak the process a bit to practice it. However, pregnant women should not practice intermittent fasting at all in any form until they have given birth to the child and stopped feeding the child with breast milk. A pregnant woman has very high energy needs. She has to eat for two lives and even store continuously. Restricting diet at such a stage, or remaining hungry for long can have serious repercussions on the mental and physical health of the mother and the child.

## Breastfeeding Mothers

If you are breastfeeding your child, then you should wait a little longer before you can begin intermittent fasting. It can cause severe energy crunch, as your body needs a lot of calories. You would need to eat at frequent intervals at this stage, and hence, intermittent fasting can be a very bad idea for you.

## People with History of Eating Disorders

For obvious reasons, if you have ever had eating disorders, you shouldn't follow intermittent fasting, as that can trigger the same problems once again if they have subsided. Intermittent fasting can cause a severe nutrient deficiency in such people.

## People with Type 1 Diabetes

People with type 1 diabetes should never practice intermittent fasting or fasting of any type for that matter. You would need to eat at regular intervals to maintain a healthy blood sugar level, and hence, you should completely avoid intermittent fasting.

## Chronically Stressed People

Chronic stress can be a problem for a person trying to practice intermittent fasting. Food is deeply connected to our emotions and our sense of security. Prolonged deprivation of food may lead to mood swings and other similar problems. People with such a condition should avoid intermittent fasting.

## People with Sleep Disorders

The toughest phase of intermittent fasting passes away while you are sleeping. If you have any kind of sleep disorder, then the chances are that it may get intensified due to the extra load of hunger pangs and food cravings. It may also affect your satisfaction levels. People facing such disorders should avoid fasting.

# Chapter 17: Getting the Best Out of Intermittent Fasting Routine

To get the best out of intermittent fasting routine, you will need to follow the 4 golden rules:

## Proper Nutrition

Food plays a very important role in your health, and it also plays an equally important role in keeping you fit. Most people are attracted towards intermittent fasting as they believe that it doesn't put any limits on food items. This is only one way to look at things. Intermittent fasting simply doesn't ask you to ban any specific type of food as that exercise only leads to a buildup of temptation and negative attitude towards the process. However, you will have to maintain a routine in which your food will have to be in accordance with your health and weight loss goals. You can't simply keep dumping soda cans into your body and expect your weight to go down anytime soon.

Your weight loss would be proportional to the kind of food you have. If you take a high-fat low-carb diet, the ketosis process can begin fast, and you will lose fast. Whereas, if you stick to a normal sugar-rich diet, it may take very long for you to get results.

There is no doubt in the fact that intermittent fasting will help you even if you don't change your diet and stick to a carb-rich diet. The process will still help you in dealing with the issue of insulin resistance and all the other associated problems. However, burning fat would remain slow in this case.

You must only expect progress in the amount of effort you are ready to put in the process.

## Healthy Exercise Routine

A healthy exercise routine is very important for faster weight loss. One of the biggest reasons for most health issues is the lack of ample physical activity. Our lives have got mechanized to a great extent. We have cars for traveling, and hence we don't need to walk. We have machines for harvesting, and hence producing food is also not a very labor-intensive job. We get readymade clothes. We can get pretty much everything done through machines. This makes most people a couch potato. They start leading a sedentary life. Their energy expenditure goes down considerably. To lose fat and weight, you will have to work hard. A healthy exercise routine is the only way you are going to get that level of activity in your life.

If you are sincere about weight loss and health, you must develop a routine for exercise. There is nothing else that can help you in burning calories faster. Start slowly with easy exercise and keep increasing the time and level of your exercise slowly.

This way, you will be able to get better and faster benefits of intermittent fasting.

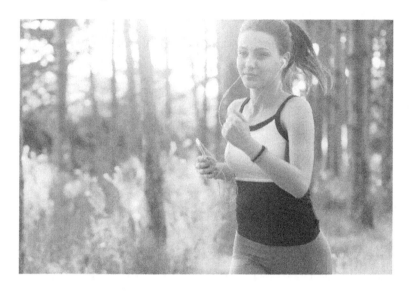

## Optimum Sleep

Most people undermine the importance of rest and sleep in good health. You must give due importance to both these things. You must sleep for 7-8 hours every day. Our body does a lot of repair and maintenance work in sleep, and hence, proper sleep is vital. You must also not try to push your body harder beyond the physical limits. Giving the body the required rest is very important. You must take at least one day gap between High-Intensity Interval Training days. Doing HIIT without giving your body the required rest can make the recovery of the body difficult. A lot of muscles get damaged during exercise, which need time to regenerate. If you won't give them the time, your progress would always be slow and erratic.

Give your body the required rest. Do not push it beyond limits. Try to sleep as much as possible.

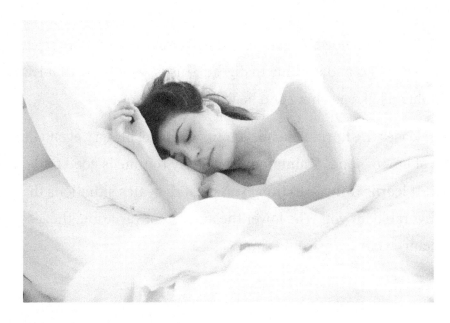

## Maintain a Routine

Maintaining a healthy routine is very important. As I have been stressing from the very beginning of the book; if you are not able to follow a routine, this process of intermittent fasting wouldn't remain sustainable. The more often you break your routine, the harder it will get for your body to adjust to the change.

For instance, our gut releases a hormone called Ghrelin. The function of this hormone is to create hunger pangs and trigger the release of gastric juices. Our body releases this hormone as clockwork. If you are habitual of eating food at a particular time, your body will release the ghrelin hormone around that time only.

This saves you from the troubles of unnecessary hunger pangs. However, if you maintain an erratic eating pattern, it would become very difficult for your body to judge the exact time to release the hormone.

If it releases the hormone early, you will have the excessive release of gastric juices and nothing to digest. This is something that leads to problems like belching and heartburn.

If it releases the hormone late, you may not feel hungry even at the time of having food. Maintaining a healthy routine is good for your body. It learns from everything you do and creates situations that are favorable for you. The lower the amount of variation, the less resistance your body would show.

# Chapter 18: Setting Milestones

Good health is an endless journey. As long as we are alive, good health should always remain our goal. However, when we start our journey towards good health, it is always important to set milestones to gauge our progress.

Milestones help in judging the progress, and also give us an insight for course correction.

Unlike other weight loss measures, intermittent fasting is not linear. It has a wide scope. People practice intermittent fasting for various objectives.

People follow intermittent fasting for 3 main purposes:

1.  Losing Weight and Burning Fat
2.  Maintaining the Current Weight
3.  Holistic Health

You can be practicing intermittent fasting for any of these goals, but you can't judge the progress with the same scale. It is important that you set benchmarks for progress to ensure that the methods are working for you.

Your goals must also be in line with the kind of effort you are putting in. If you are putting in a lot of effort, and yet you are not getting the results, then you would need to do course correction.

# Intermittent Fasting for Burning Fat and Losing Weight

This is one of the most popular goals, as people these days are really struggling with weight issues.

There are two ways to judge progress in this area.

1. You should measure the target areas like the waistline, hips, and thighs with a measuring tape to see if the fat burning is taking place.
2. You should weigh yourself on the scale to see if the weight is going down.

There can be anyone of the following scenarios:

a. *Your weight is going down, but your waistline remains the same*
This happens in the first few weeks of beginning intermittent fasting. Your weight may drop drastically as the body starts dumping a lot of water. You must have patience as the body would start burning fat very soon.

b. *You are losing weight as well as your waistline is also going down*
This usually happens in the beginning phases, and your body loses weight as well as it burns fat too.

c. *Your waistline is going down, but your weight is not going down*
This can happen when your body burns fat, but also starts building muscles. The muscles are compact and have more

weight. Therefore, you may not see any significant change in your weight on the scale. However, this is a positive thing.

If your observation is something different, then you would need to revisit the whole process and determine the point where you are making a deviation of mistake.

# Intermittent Fasting for Weight Maintenance

Maintenance of the existing weight is also a goal people have these days, and it is a very important thing. If the weight starts growing uncontrollably, the day is not far when you will be surrounded by a number of diseases. Therefore, it is important that you get a weight bracket for yourself.

You can make changes in your diet and workout routines whenever you notice any significant change in your weight bracket or the waistline.

# Intermittent Fasting for Improving Overall Health

Improvement of overall health is a goal everyone must have. If you are healthy, the accumulation of fat is the last thing to happen. Your body is always capable of fighting all the excesses. To judge improvement in health, you will need to take some tests before beginning intermittent fasting, and then keep repeating them at regular intervals.

# Chapter 19: Staying Motivated

Remaining motivated on the path of weight loss can be tough or challenging at times. Losing weight is a lonely road. People may praise you for the improvements you make, but no one is there to share your trials and tribulations. The pains and gains of the weight loss journey always stay with you.

Weight loss journeys can be really disappointing and painful at times. There may come times when you would want to put your guard down. There are points of disillusionment in the life of almost everyone passing through this journey where he/she starts feeling the whole process futile and worthless. It is not the journey that becomes worthless; it is our mind trying to find an excuse to get out of the tough situation. It is simply a reaction of fight or flight response.

You must stay strong and motivated. These times are painful, but they pass away very quickly. You must draw inspiration from people around you, and take support from the people near and dear to you.

The best way to survive and thrive on this path is to find your support pillars. You can draw support from the following:

# Friends and Family

This is the natural support base for everyone. It is a reliable support base you can look up to. It is important that you confide in them as it gives you power. You are able to share your victories and failures with them, and hence, nothing keeps building inside you. You will always find yourself as light as a feather.

Sharing your problems or challenges with family and friends also helps in avoiding uncomfortable situations. If you are trying to avoid eating a certain type of food, the family members can avoid bringing or eating it in front of you. The atmosphere remains more empathetic.

# Support Groups

You find people suffering from the same problems in support groups, and hence, you are able to relate to them and share your problems with them easily. Support groups play a great role in removing inhibitions. People don't feel strange, and they are better able to answer each other's questions. Most people have been through similar situations, hence, it is easier to find people with common struggles.

# Professionals

You can also take the help of professionals like doctors, dieticians, nutritionists. They are better equipped to answer your technical queries, and they can guide you in the right direction. If you are already suffering from any chronic illness, then you must seek the help of a professional; as regular monitoring of the problem is important for your very own safety.

# Conclusion

Thank you for making it through to the end of this book, let's hope it was informative and able to provide you with all the tools you need to achieve your goals; whatever they may be.

16/8 intermittent fasting is an easy to follow method of losing weight. It takes you on a clear-cut path to not only lose weight, but also helps you in burning a lot of fat in the body.

This intermittent fasting technique is specifically designed to provide holistic health benefits, and would ensure that you lead a healthy and active life.

This biggest advantage of this intermittent fasting technique is that it is very simple and easy to follow. You can practice it irrespective of the life you live or work you do. It will be suitable for you if you have a desk job, and equally helpful even if your line of business requires a lot of traveling.

It would work seamlessly for a stay at home mom, and would work wonders for a working woman with a hectic work life. With a little bit of dedication and discipline, anyone can make this plan work for himself/herself.

You can also get all the benefits of the process by following the simple steps given in the book. I hope that this book is really able to help you in achieving your health goals.

Finally, if you found this book useful in any way, a review on Amazon is always appreciated!

# Book 2: One Meal a Day

*A scientific method for quick and healthy weight loss.*

*A step-by-step guide that will help you increase mental clarity, rejuvenate your energy, and reduce inflammation.*

**By Rose Heale**

# Introduction

Congratulations on choosing this book and thank you for doing so. This book will help you in understanding the amazing concept of One Meal a Day routine and the way it can help you in burning fat and improving your overall health.

Obesity and associated health problems have become a major concern these days. Modern lifestyle, poor eating habits, and unhealthy food items have contributed greatly to the problem.

Reducing weight is a difficult process and the weight relapse is generally much faster than weight loss. Therefore, after months of hard work in the gym and restrictive eating through diet plans, we find ourselves standing back to square one.

The weight loss industry is thriving as more and more people are facing the problem of obesity yet very few people can honestly say that they have truly benefitted from the procedures.

One Meal a Day is a routine through which you can break the jinx of weight relapse. You will be able to lose weight and burn fat effectively. This is a process through which losing weight wouldn't remain an impossible task.

To some, One Meal a Day in itself may look like an impossible task. Staying away from food for such a long period every day may look scary and unimaginable. However, it isn't such a difficult task as it sounds. One Meal a Day is a scientific process of systematic conditioning of the body. You wouldn't have to start fasting for the whole day for the very beginning. There will be steps and a slow transition to the final process.

This book will help you in understanding the science behind One Meal a Day routine and the easy ways through which you can successfully incorporate it into your life.

This book will also explain all the health benefits that come along with this routine and the ways in which it can make your life easier.

It will serve as a guide to understand the process completely and the right way to follow it for great success. You would also get to know the specific challenges that you may face and the ways to deal with those challenges.

This book will also give you a comparative analysis of other weight loss methods and the scientific reasons behind their failure and also why One Meal a Day routine can easily overcome those challenges.

This book will help you in not only losing weight and burning fat but also staying healthier. It will explain the dangers you might be facing due to excess weight and the ways to get over them.

One of the biggest challenges people face is not only to lose weight but also to maintain it. Most weight loss procedures tell you the ways to shed a few pounds but they have no way to maintain that way for the long term. The reason behind this failure is the problem in maintaining those procedures as a daily routine.

One Meal a Day routine wins over them in this race. It is a lifestyle change that you can incorporate and easily ensure that the weight you lose never comes back.

This book will guide you about healthy ways to stay fit and healthy. It will explain all this to you in easy and simple steps.

With plenty of books written on the subject, we would thank you for getting this book! Every effort was made to ensure it is full of as much useful information as possible, please enjoy!

# Part I

## Chapter 1: Obesity- A Simple Overview

# Obesity - The Facts

Obesity is a curse of the modern age, poor lifestyle, and bad eating habits. There was a time it was solely considered to be a problem of the affluent and developed world, but times have changed lately. Obesity has emerged as a global epidemic in the past four decades affecting the rich and poor alike.

WHO report of 2016 states that worldwide obesity rates have tripled since 1975. In the year 2016, more than 1.9 billion adults were overweight or obese. However, a major portion of this number comes from the developed world.

As a matter of fact, more than 71.6% of the US adult population is battling with this weight management issues. The problem is equally widespread in Europe and other regions. Although resentfully, the developed world has accepted the problem as it is clearly evident and undeniably obvious. Most people have realized that there is no point sticking the neck in the sand. Still, a lot of people try to pass the buck on a fast-paced lifestyle, hectic work life, stress, lack of time to pay attention to health and several such things, but a large part of the population has also been trying earnestly and furiously to deal with the problem. However, the results have been far and few between.

What has emerged as more shocking news to the world is the fact that over 340 million children falling in the age group of 5-16 were also found to be overweight or obese during the same period. This is a group that was not exposed to the above-mentioned problems in that severity. This makes it evident that although these may be contributing facts to obesity, they are not the sole reasons. The problem is severe and it is growing at an exponential rate. If not dealt with properly, it can pose a big threat even for our future generations.

The current stats show that more than 2 out of 3 American adults are overweight. Almost 39.8% of the US adult population is suffering from obesity with a BMI range higher than 30. Primarily, obesity may look like a cosmetic issue but it has far serious consequences.

Obesity is a chronic medical disease. It is difficult to treat and has a very high relapse rate. The biggest problem with obesity is that it doesn't come alone. It hunts in a pack. It unleashes the wrath of several debilitating conditions like diabetes, cholesterol problem, hypertension, and other metabolic issues. A person facing obesity becomes prone to a score of problems.

## The Problem

The biggest problem with obesity has been its treatment. It is hard to treat. The increase in weight itself makes losing weight difficult. Several metabolic issues hover around the victim and pose hurdles in losing weight. Diseases like heart conditions, diabetes, and hypertension make heavy exercise and other weight loss measures difficult.

People resort to various short term weight loss measures like dieting, rigorous exercise, medication, and surgery but they also largely show inconsistent results. Most people who use these short term fixes for obesity regain the original weight or more within 5 years.

Obesity and the problems arising with it have started raising great concerns among people. One of the most common conditions associated with obesity is the blood sugar control problem that later turns into prediabetes and diabetes . It is currently affecting more than 110 million US adults. People suffering from high-cholesterol issues are in even greater numbers and the same goes for people suffering from hypertension. Obesity and the problems associated with it are among the top 5 major causes leading to preventable deaths in the US. Out of the 900,000 preventable deaths recorded in the US every year almost 40% have these issues in the list.

People want to get rid of the problems and they look towards weight loss measures. This has given rise to the weight loss industry. The market value of the weight loss industry in the US alone is a whopping $72 billion. If you also count the market value of the weight loss industry in Europe too, the figure may rise to hundreds of billions. It is interesting to note that the weight loss industry is very new and has emerged in the past few decades only. However, the troublesome fact is that although on one side the weight loss industry is registering a year on year growth, on the other side, the obesity rates are also rising consistently. Therefore, it is evident that even after spending billions of dollars on weight loss every year, the obesity rates are not going down.

The weight loss industry is always eager to push new methods, fad diets, wonder pills and surgical methods to treat obesity. It is always optimistic in its tone and fervor until you enroll. Like any other industry, it works on financial motivation. However, it always has an advantage, it can always push the blame on you. It is the only industry in the world which conveniently blames the customers for its failures and you would have no other choice than to take the blame and shame.

The industry mainly focuses on quick fixes and instant results to justify the costs. However, obesity is a chronic problem and so, it's either nothing happens at all or the lost weight comes back very soon. It is a problem that develops through ignorance of years and hence curing it in a short span of time isn't possible or practical.

## **The Solution**

The real problem lies in the understanding of weight gain. All these methods have the ability to bring down weight. Even your body has the ability to remain slim and fit without any external help. This is evident from the fact that although humankind has been on this earth for thousands of years, obesity is a fairly new world problem. Our body has been successfully fighting weight issues for a very long period and it can still do the same under the right conditions. However, we are not able to provide the right environment to our body to shed the weight due to our ignorance and indiscipline.

You can easily lose weight through any of the weight loss methods if your body stops acting against you. But, that never happens or it would be correct to say that you never allow your body to do the same because you are always sending the wrong signals to your system.

While you are trying to burn fat, your body is constantly receiving the message to store fat. This works against you and losing weight remains a bleak possibility. Even if there are some results they are mostly short-lived and inconsistent.

This book is going to help you to understand the real reasons for the problem and the ways to resolve them. This is your guide not only for losing weight and burning the adamant fat deposits but also for achieving holistic health through some simple yet effective methods.

Losing weight doesn't involve doing something extra but avoiding things that are bad. This book will help you in understanding the ways through which you can bring the change in your body by bringing a bit of discipline in your life without adding anything extra to it.

This book will help you in understanding the reasons for the increasing rate of obesity in a step by step manners and the ways we can counter it. The biggest problem in any weight loss routine is sticking to the routine on a long-term basis. This book will help you in figuring out the ways in which you can make that happen.

This book will not ask you to do something out of ordinary as it is not possible to follow extraordinary routines in the fast-paced life driven by cut-throat competition and impending deadlines. It lays down a very practical and easy roadmap for you to follow so that you can break the obesity jinx.

## Body Mass Index

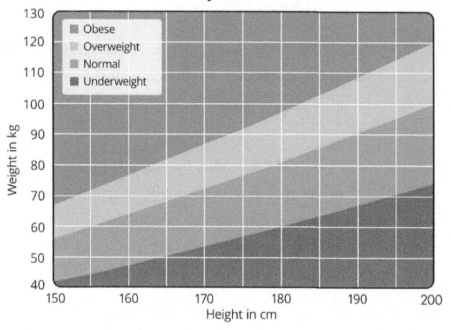

# Chapter 2: Fat Burning Mechanism

We all understand that obesity is a problem. The simple calculation of calories is also fed to us through all channels. Most people believe that it is as simple as that. However, the problem is that it isn't that simple.

Let's suppose that you lead a sedentary life with low physical activity. It is a sad reality for most of us as there is stiff competition and most of us have to slog longer hours to remain relevant in the market. This means that the number of calories you burn in a day are few in comparison to a person who has a physically active life.

If you are burning 2500 calories a day in your daily routine then according to popular math if you start consuming 2000 calories it will create a deficit of 500 calories. Your body needs 2500 calories but you are supplying less. Ideally, your body should start using the stored fat for fulfilling the deficit of 500 calories. This means you should lose weight. This is where you and your body differ.

## Our Body's Treatment of Fat

The fat in the body has some very important functions. Fat is stored energy. Our body stores fat for survival in tough times. It is the reserve fuel for the times when you will have no energy supply from outside. The fat also has some other functions like hormones production, insulation of organs and absorption of nutrients. However, we will discuss that later to avoid confusion.

Our body doesn't treat fat as a problem. In fact, it treats fat as an energy reserve. Therefore, it would always try to store fat. On average, men should have 11-15% of body fat and women should have 21-25% of body fat. A woman's body is more likely to store fat as it also has an added responsibility of bearing a child. A lower fat ratio can also cause problems.

## Energy for Metabolic Functions

Our body needs a fixed number of calories for running the body. These calories are needed for running the basic body functions like pumping your heart, regulating breathing, waste excretion, and other such vital functions. You need a certain number of calories even if you do not undertake any kind of physical activity at all. It means that even if you don't get out of your bed for 2 days, the calorie needs of your body would go down but they wouldn't stop. The number of calories burnt in such condition is called the Basal Metabolic Rate or (BMR).

So, if your BMR is 2000 and you do some physical activity like going to the office and burn 500 calories in the process, your calorie requirement would be 2500. Therefore, it looks obvious that if you reduce the calorie intake by 500 calories your body would have to compensate the deficit from somewhere.

Alas! That doesn't happen in normal conditions.

Body's Way of Compensating the Loss of Calories

Life started on this planet millions of years ago. We have evolved into a complex multicellular organism from single cellular life forms. This means passing through the evolutionary process for millions of years. Tricking the body to fall for this deceit is difficult and that's what happens.

As soon as you lower the calorie intake, the body registers the shortfall. It triggers the survival mechanism and your body starts lowering the metabolic rate to match the deficit. This means that when you lower your calorie intake your BMR also goes down. You start consuming fewer calories and your body would match for the loss and stop burning calories extensively.

If you have ever been in any kind of calorie restrictive-diet, you must have noticed that the body starts feeling lethargic. You don't feel like doing anything much. You get tired early. You start feeling fatigued very often. You don't feel like doing things. You get irritated very fast. You start having mood swings. All these are signals from your body that the metabolic rate has gone slower.

This means that by consuming fewer calories, you are not going to gain much.

But, You or Your Friend Lost Weight

It is very much possible for people to rapidly lose some weight. However, **there is no light at the end of the tunnel.**

Remember we talked about some other functions of fat in our body other than providing energy. One of the functions is to provide insulation. Our body generally stores a lot of water in order to maintain body temperature and provide insulation. A high portion of the calories consumed by you on a daily basis is used for providing this insulation. It keeps you warm in winters and also saves you from unbearable heat.

However, as soon as you lower your calorie intake, the body starts looking for an efficient way to manage the deficit. The first thing it does is dump the excess water to conserve energy. So, there is a lot of fluid loss at the beginning of calorie restrictive diets. This loss of fluids gets registered as loss of weight on the scale and you get a false notion that you are actually losing weight or burning fat.

Here, it is important that this fluid loss is not permanent and as soon as you would resume a normal diet, the body would again try to maintain a comfortable temperature and water retention would begin. This is a reason for rapidly gaining weight after getting off diets.

Diets are also restrictive in nature and people are often get tempted into binge eating and that also contributes heavily towards rapid weight gain.

Losing a few pounds on the scale is not the right measure of success. **You must also lose a few inches of belly fat or fat on your thighs and hips** and that would be the right way to measure success.

# Fat Burning Mechanism

Our body has a very sophisticated energy mechanism. There are energy backup structures to ensure that you survive the longest. The fat is a savior for your body and not an enemy.

The food you eat doesn't get stored as fat directly. All the excess food that you eat wouldn't get stored as fat. All the fat in your body isn't that bad.

The Process of Storing Energy

Anything that you eat gets converted into calories. These calories are then dumped into your bloodstream where they get processed at various levels.

Let's first understand the three levels of energy storage:

1. **Glucose:** Whatever you eat is released into your blood in the form of glucose. It is the simplest form of energy your cells can absorb directly.
   a. Your body loves to use glucose as it is easy to process.
   b. As soon as glucose is mixed into your bloodstream your blood sugar levels rise.
   c. The pancreas in the body senses the heightened blood sugar level and releases '**Insulin**' hormone for stabilizing it.
   d. Insulin is a very important hormone as it not only helps in the absorption of glucose it is also the main fat-storage hormone.

e. The insulin works as the key to allow the glucose absorption by the cells.

f. Insulin attaches itself to the cells and facilitates the absorption of glucose.

g. However, the cells can't absorb all the glucose, they have very limited storage ability.

2. **Glycogen:** If the blood sugar levels in your body still remain high after the cells have absorbed all the required glucose the insulin starts trying to adjust the levels by storing it in secondary form. This secondary storage is in the form of Glycogen.

   **a.** Glycogen gets stored primarily in the muscles and the liver.

   **b.** The muscles can also store glycogen in limited quantity as the energy stored here can only be used by that particular muscle.

   **c.** One muscle can't transfer this energy stored in the form glycogen to another muscle in times of need.

   **d.** It is strictly for personal use. This is the energy you use while running or doing any other physical activity.

   **e.** A big part of glycogen gets stored in the liver as it has the ability to use it for producing glucose for cells when needed.

   **f.** This is the energy store your body would be using first whenever it is short of ready energy supply.

3. **Fat:** This is the final energy storage point and here any amount of energy can be stored. If the blood sugar level still remains high even after storing glycogen in the muscles and liver, insulin would signal the fat cells to store the remaining energy as fat. This is the most stubborn kind of fat that just doesn't go.

   a. It is the job of the insulin to signal the fat cells to store the remaining glucose as fat

   b. The adipose tissues store the excess glucose as subcutaneous fat. This is the belly fat or fat deposited at the thighs and muscles.

   c. This fat make certain people feel that they look unattractive but it is generally not very harmful.

   d. These are just the jiggly fat deposits on your belly, thigh, and hips.

   e. However, if there is excess fat in your body it starts covering your internal organs as visceral fat.

   f. This is the most dangerous fat as it can cause several chronic problems including inflammations.

   g. Visceral fat is the most difficult to lose and causes most of the problems in your body.

   h. It is the fat responsible for diseases like:

      i. Type II diabetes

      ii. Hypertension

      iii. Heart disorders

      iv. Hormonal imbalance

      v. Stroke

vi.    Breast and Colorectal Cancer

vii.    Alzheimer's disease

viii.    Insulin resistance

Therefore, burning visceral fat is the most important task and it is also the most difficult one. Your body doesn't accumulate visceral fat overnight and would never start burning it first.

If you want to burn the visceral fat in your body and stay healthy, it is important that you take the right steps.

The Problem with Conventional Fat Burning Methods

All fat burning methods are principally correct in theory. If you consume less and burn more, your body would not have any other option than to burn the fat stored.

However, there are problems with this idea:

1. When you start doing aggressive physical exercise or activity, the energy in your cells gets spent first. The cells stores a very limited amount of energy and hence you easily reach the second energy store.

2. The energy stored in the form of glycogen in muscles and liver is the second energy source.

3. Glycogen stored in the liver can provide energy for about 24 hours after your last meal.

4. Only after the glycogen stores are depleted and your energy demands are still high your fat stores would metabolize.

# The Conclusion

The real problem with fat burning is creating a deficit of energy. Till now we have understood that our body has plenty of energy stores. It will first use the blood glucose, then the glycogen and finally begin using the fat for energy.

The glucose in the cells lasts for a few hours but the glycogen in your liver can last for 24 hours from your last meal. This means that even if you have a small meal within this period, the whole process will begin again. Even a few calories consumed can refuel your body and it would focus more on energy conservation rather than energy-burning as it would be counterintuitive in terms of survival strategy.

Another Big Problem- Insulin

Insulin, as we have already discussed, is a very important hormone that plays a very crucial role in energy storage and lowering our blood glucose levels. We also know that it is the main fat-storage hormone and that is also a big part of the problem in weight loss efforts.

Before we begin understanding insulin and the problems associated with it let us try to understand the situation through an analogy.

Suppose you are in your office and there is a lot of pending work in your office. Your immediate boss whose sits across is getting on your nerves to clear all the files on your desk before you can go out to meet your friend waiting for you outside your office.

Your friend is getting impatient and he is messaging you incessantly and causing distraction. Some of your coworkers at the coffee maker are also having a very interesting conversation that you want to be a part of. However, the problem is that although there may not be any restriction to go to the pantry and move around in the office, you can't leave until you finish the work. Your boss doesn't like you roaming around in the office and every time you make a trip to the coffee machine, the boss gets miffed and increases your workload.

You are caught in the middle of a problem:

1. You can't leave the office and meet your friend although you want to as your work is not finished.
2. Until your boss is there, you can't go. The boss wouldn't leave the office until you submit the work.
3. You can go to the pantry anytime as you want but that again would keep you tied to your office even longer.
4. Your friend is constantly messaging and you are feeling irritated.

These things get you in an uncomfortable position to be. However, there are times when we know the problem and its solution but can't quite figure out the way to get out of it.

The same is the case with the **INSULIN PROBLEM**

# The Boss

As we know insulin is the main fat-storage hormone. As long as insulin is present in your bloodstream, there can be no fat burning in your body. If you try to burn more calories than you have consumed, you will start feeling tired. The reason is simple, insulin will prevent any kind of fat burning. You are forced to work out with what you have. There can be no excuse. In the above analogy, insulin is the boss.

## The Pantry

Our eating patterns have changed drastically in the past few decades. The food industry has moved ahead leaps and bounds making it possible to store unlimited quantities of ready to eat food in our fridges. The abundance of food all around brought to us by food security due to modern farming techniques that have made it very easy and affordable to buy food. This has increased the number of times we eat in a day. Including snacks, we have 5-8 meals on a usual day. If you even start counting the beverages and munchies that we have, this number can go much higher.

The problem is that after every meal, howsoever insignificant, your pancreas releases insulin to lower the blood sugar levels. Once the insulin is released, it takes at least 8-12 hours for the insulin levels to dissipate. This means the higher the number of meals you have or the shorter the interval between your meals, the lower would be the probability of insulin levels ever getting low. It would also mean that your body would never come in the fat-burning mode in real terms.

In our analogy, the frequent meals are the coworkers at the coffee machine in the pantry. The more frequently you visit them, the longer it would take you to finish the work. It would also mean that you wouldn't be able to go out to meet your friend.

These days snacking or frequently having beverages like tea, coffee, shakes, soda, etc. has become a trend. We all like to keep our selves hydrated and these items also help us in focusing. But, this is all an illusion. The refreshing feeling that you get after munching on the wafers, chips, and chocolates or sipping your favorite beverage is because of the relieving effect of addiction that these things have on our body. These things are not helping our system but overloading it with calories and the sugar and carbs in these things are adding to the problem.

## The Friend

The friend waiting for you outside is your health. The longer you remain indulged in this lifestyle the more difficult it would become for you to get out of the trap of obesity. Exercise, dieting, and all other such weight loss measures are the smart work that you can do to finish your work fast. They can help you in getting out of the office fast. But, nothing would happen until you stop getting distracted by the coworkers at the coffee machine. The more frequently you visit them, the more work your boss would keep giving you.

The only way to get out of this trap is to avoid the pantry and focus on your work. Most diets focus on reducing the calorie intake but they ignore the real fat burning mechanism in the body. The body wouldn't start burning fat until there is insulin floating around in high quantities in your bloodstream and that would remain a problem as long as you keep having frequent meals or keep ingesting calories through beverages.

## Problem Computation

The real problem with fat burning is our lifestyle and poor eating habits. We have made frequent eating a lifestyle. There is an abundance of food all around us and we have also started treating food casually. Most people believe that they can remain healthy by simply eating healthy food. Some don't even care about healthy food. In both cases, our health suffers greatly.

Counting calories alone is not going to help you in losing weight as your body would never really be in a position to burn weight. A high presence of insulin would always keep your body in fat-storage mode and the body would find itself unable to start burning fat.

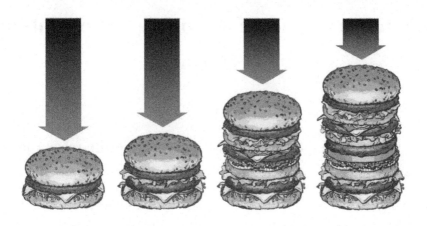

If you want to burn fat that bringing a complete change in your eating habits is mandatory and then only any real benefit of weight loss can be experienced. One Meal A Day routine can help you in this process greatly. It deals with the problem of the excessive presence of insulin in your bloodstream. The longer the interval between meals, the easier it would become for your body to start the fat burning mechanism.

# Chapter 3: Impact of Changing Eating Pattern on Obesity

In the previous chapter, we tried to understand the reason for the failure of most weight loss measures and the mechanism of fat burning. The first and foremost requirement for fat burning in the body is the absence of insulin in the bloodstream.

Insulin is an important fat-storage hormone that our pancreas releases every time we consume calories. Frequent meals decrease the probability of fat burning in the body.

An Overview of the Historical Eating Patterns

Our eating patterns have changed drastically in the past few centuries. Historically speaking, gathering food was always difficult. We began as hunter-gatherers. Therefore, finding food was always difficult. Our ancestors never got food in abundance. They had to toil very hard to get food. It involved intense physical activity as well as luck. The odds of getting food were less. Getting one good meal a day was fortunate enough. This is a reason people may have died of several reasons but obesity wasn't among them.

Then, we shifted to agriculture. It increased the probability of getting food but still, the situation was nothing like the current era. Cultivating food was still a labor intensive job and hence we were burning more calories in the process than we were consuming and hence the overall health of the general population remained robust.

The current age has brought great sophistication in food production technology. Getting food has become easy and less labor intensive. The food is also comparatively cheap and hence people can easily afford it. This has given rise to abuse of food. We are not eating as per our needs but as per our desires.

Our body has evolved through millions of years in a food-starved environment. It likes to store energy. The mechanism is built in such a way that storing energy gives a sense of security. However, it is acting against our body as our intake has increased manifolds but the expenditure has gone down considerably. The labor-intensive jobs are carried out through machines and hence we have to rely more on exercises for burning calories.

This change in our eating pattern has led to problems that can only be resolved by addressing the underlying issues in food consumption patterns.

To burn fat there are some simple requirements:

- You must give your body the right conditions to facilitate fat burning
- You must consume less and burn more calories
- You have to make sure you check what you eat

If you can fulfill these three simple conditions, burning fat and maintaining the lost weight would become very easy and simple.

One Meal a Day is an easy way to fulfill all the three conditions without going an extra mile in your daily life.

# Conditions Facilitating Fat Burning

As we have understood, fat burning is a complex process. The basic requirement of fat burning is that your body must not be in a fat-storage mode. This will not happen until there is a high-presence of insulin in your blood.

When you begin practicing the One Meal a Day routine, frequent consumption of calories comes to a stop. One meal a day means that you will only supply the required calories to your body only once a day. Processing that meal and absorption of blood sugar would take another 8-12 hour. However, after this time, the insulin levels in your bloodstream would go down considerably as there will be no blood sugar spike. You will not be supplying more glucose to your body during this period.

This creates the required energy deficit. Your body has no other option than to begin using the energy reserves. The glucose stored in the cells lasts only for a few hours. Your body feels the need for energy and hence the liver starts metabolizing its glycogen stores. Fully replenished glycogen stores can last for 24 hours. However, when you start following One Meal a Day routine your general calorie intake gets limited. There isn't excess energy to replenish the glycogen stores like before. Therefore, soon your glycogen stores wouldn't last even that long and hence your body would have no other option than to begin metabolization of the fat stores.

# Consuming Less and Burning More

When you start following One Meal a Day routine, your calorie consumption rate goes down. This routine generally doesn't restrict your calorie intake. However, as you can only have one meal in a day, consuming too many calories in a single meal always remains a challenge. Therefore, calorie control comes automatically. You don't need to count the calories anymore. You are always free to consume as much food as you can within a reasonable limit. You can treat yourself with the food of your choice as long as it is healthy.

Your calorie consumption goes down and your body begins burning more calories as the BMR remains the same.

Here, you can have the doubt that wouldn't the BMR go down when the calorie intake is low.

The answer to that is NO.

When you begin dieting, you are consuming food at regular intervals but the calorie intake gets low. The body goes in survival mode as it is noticing a consistent reduction in calories. That doesn't happen when you are following One Meal a Day routine.

The single meal of your day will be providing calories in ample quantity and hence the body wouldn't feel the need to lower the BMR.

The times when your body needs more energy and it isn't getting any regular supply, there will be no insulin present in your blood. Therefore, your body would be in a position to start metabolization of the fat stores for making up for the energy deficit. Our body has an ample amount of fat to run the body for months without food. Running it for a few hours would not trigger any kind of survival mechanism.

Eating the Right Kind of Food

Food plays a very important role in our health. It also affects our eating habits and food cravings. If you are eating a carbohydrate-rich diet, it will load your system with instant calories. However, it would also create food cravings very fast. The same goes for sugar-rich foods. These things will make controlling hunger very difficult. Going without food for a very long period on such a diet would become very difficult for you.

On the other hand, if you start consuming a balanced diet with the right mix of fat, proteins, and carbs, it would become very easy for you to control your food cravings. A balanced diet also provides the required nutrients and gives your gut the right environment to facilitate good health.

One Meal a Day routine can help you in losing weight and burning fat. It helps your body in fighting the problems that have been created by frequent abuse of food that has been taking place for years.

It may sound difficult as staying on a simple meal for the whole day may sound like a very demanding thing. However, this book will explain in detail the ways in which you can follow this routine easily and it wouldn't sound as drastic as it feels.

It is important to understand that changing eating patterns is the only reliable way to manage weight and body fat effectively. It is a way your body knows very well. It would not only help you in losing weight and burning fat but would also help you in improving overall health biomarkers. You will feel healthier, rejuvenated, and full of energy.

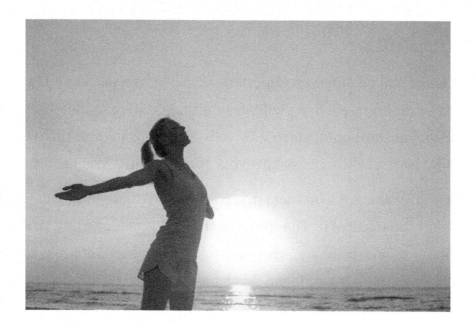

# Chapter 4: One Meal A Day- Game Changer for Fat Burning

Until now, we have mostly discussed the issues prohibiting fat burning. We have also discussed the role of insulin in the whole fat burning scenario. Before we move ahead to the next section and discuss the ways in which One Meal a Day routine can bring a holistic change in your life, it is important that you also understand one major problem that is causing most of the health issues.

## Insulin Resistance- Mother of All Problems

We know that insulin is an important hormone. We also know that it is the main hormone that facilitates the stabilization of blood sugar level and absorption of glucose by cells. But, do you know that your current eating habits are making your body insulin resistant.

Insulin resistance is a problem that plagues most of us but we remain blissfully unaware of it. The reason is that it doesn't have any visible symptoms and it remains a chronic problem that keeps eroding your body. However, it is a problem that leads to most of the health issues we face in our day to day lives.

Diabetes, hypertension, fatty liver disease, heart problems, fat accumulation, metabolic disorders, and many other such diseases are a direct consequence of this nasty condition that is caused by our erratic eating habits.

172

# What is Insulin Resistance

Insulin resistance is a condition in which your cells stop responding actively to the signals of insulin and don't open up to receive glucose. This may not sound that scary but it is a bigger problem than most of the problems you may know.

High blood sugar levels are dangerous for your body. If your blood sugar levels start remaining consistently high then it can lead to thickening of vessels in your vital organs. It can make them stiff and affect their functionality. That's why, as soon as your blood sugar level goes up, the pancreas in the body starts pumping insulin into your bloodstream so that the blood sugar levels can be managed fast.

Your cells also need a regular supply of glucose for maintaining their functionality. However, if their ability to bind with insulin goes down, they wouldn't be able to receive glucose and would starve. Therefore, it is important that insulin sensitivity remains good.

# How Does Insulin Resistance Develop

Insulin resistance is a condition that develops when your cells start getting overexposure to insulin. It is like a nosy neighbor who is always sticking the nose in your doorway. One is always eager and welcoming to guests especially neighbors as long as they maintain a safe distance. But, imagine what if your neighbor starts banging your door all the time and any time of the day or night.

This happens when you eat meals at short intervals. Whenever you consume a meal or any beverage that contains calories it gets processed and converted into glucose. This glucose mixes into your bloodstream and raises the blood sugar levels. The pancreas senses the increase in blood sugar level and starts pumping insulin to stabilize the levels.

The insulin spreads across the body and knocks at the cells to enable them to receive the fresh glucose supply. However, if this process starts getting repeated very often, the cells start responding slow to the insulin signals. This means that although your body would have a high presence of insulin yet your blood sugar levels would remain high and your cells would also remain energy starved. They stop responding to the insulin signals and they can't even absorb the glucose directly without insulin.

On the other hand, the pancreas would sense the high blood sugar level and would keep pumping more and more insulin to manage the blood sugar. This even increases the problem. The cells develop insulin resistance as they are usually overexposed to the insulin hormone. This increases the overexposure. The reception gets slower and slower and the blood sugar levels remain higher for longer than usual.

High insulin presence would also mean that your body would remain unable to burn any kind of fat and would constantly keep getting the signals to store fat. Therefore, all your weight loss efforts get washed down the drain if you have insulin resistance.

# How Does One Meal A Day Help

One Meal a Day help in inducing the much-needed absence of insulin in your bloodstream. You can consume one meal in a day. This meal can be big or small as that would remain inconsequential in this respect. Let us suppose that you have your one meal of the day in the evening around 7.

Now, this meal would lead to glucose release and the pancreas would pump insulin. Normally, it takes 8-12 hours from your last meal for the insulin levels to go down in your bloodstream. This means that latest by 7 in the morning your body would have minimum levels of insulin. However, by this time, your blood sugar levels would be also low as you wouldn't be consuming a new meal anytime soon.

The cells in your body would get another 5-6 hour when there is no insulin banging at their door. This prolonged absence of insulin creates a favorable environment and the cells again start responding to the signals actively. This leads to the development of insulin sensitivity.

The greater the insulin sensitivity in your body, the better it would respond to weight management efforts. You would be able to lose weight fast and enjoy a healthier and fuller life.

Prolonged fasting is the only way to develop insulin sensitivity and lower the problem of insulin resistance in your body.

If your body is insulin sensitive, your pancreas wouldn't have to pump excessive insulin into your bloodstream and hence the insulin levels would go down faster. This will also help in beginning the fat burning mechanism faster.

Your body would come out of fat-storage mode faster every day and hence burning fat would get easier and would also get more time.

Therefore, if you want to begin fat burning, bringing down insulin resistance is a must.

Prolonged fasting is a good way to develop insulin sensitivity but that's not a practical way on a regular basis. However, One Meal a Day is a practical method currently followed by millions of people to get the benefits of good health.

One Meal a Day also has loads of other health benefits besides fat burning that will be explained in the chapters to follow. They will help you in understanding the immense health benefits of following the routine.

# Part II

# Chapter 5: Boosts HGH Production for Accelerated Fat Burning

The Human Growth Hormone (HGH) has amazing abilities. Our body produces this hormone in abundance and it literally builds our body. It aids in growth and helps in healing. If you want to build muscles fast this is the hormone to look up to. If you want to burn fat quickly, this hormone can help you like wonder. The importance of this hormone is such that bodybuilders and athletes started abusing synthetically produced HGH to a dangerous extent. It is a performance enhancing hormone that can turn tables for anyone. However, the use of synthetic HGH was banned soon.

**Some of the Benefits of HGH**

> ➤ It accelerates the burning of fat
> ➤ It helps in building muscles and promotes maintenance of muscle mass
> ➤ It also increases the stamina to do high-intensity exercises for longer
> ➤ It boosts your immune system

➤ It helps in the regulation of mood and also brings positivity

➤ It has amazing anti-aging properties

➤ It accelerates healing, growth, and repair of damaged tissues

➤ It increases your libido

➤ It also helps in increasing the production of anabolic hormones in the body

## The HGH Story

Our body produces HGH in large quantities in our growing up years as it helps in our growth. The production of HGH is very high in childhood and it reaches its peak in our teenage. However, as we cross our teens and enter into our 20's the production of HGH goes low. The reason is simple, we stop growing anymore and hence our body stops feeling the need to produce HGH in large quantities. But, the production of HGH never stops completely. Our body can produce HGH if the conditions are right.

## The Ideal Conditions for Production of HGH

• When the production of hunger hormone is high in your body

• When the presence of insulin is negligible in your body

• When you are doing intense physical activity

• When you are sleeping

• When you face an injury or go through a trauma

Fasting is one of the best ways to make your body produce HGH in large quantities. It fulfills most of the conditions required for the production of HGH.

Our body produces HGH in high quantity when you are feeling hunger. Hunger bouts are common in fasting.

The insulin levels should be low to facilitate the production of HGH. When the body is in the fasting state, insulin levels go down.

When you do intense physical exercise in the fasted state, the production and effect of HGH increases. Therefore, exercising in the fasted state can be very helpful in increasing the production of HGH. It will not only facilitate faster fat burning but will also increase your stamina so that you can exercise for longer.

The American College of Cardiology states that fasting can give a 2000% boost to HGH production in men. In women, the production of HGH can rise up to 1300%.

So, if fat burning is your aim, HGH is the main hormone and you should focus more on increasing the production of this hormone. Fasting can help you in this direction a lot.

Muscle building is another forte of this hormone. It helps in the faster metabolization of fat and also facilitates muscle building. Your body will lose fat and build muscle at the same time. This is an advantage most people can never get through any other way.

# Chapter 6: Improves Leptin Sensitivity-Amazing Appetite Control

Our body has an amazing mechanism to regulate hunger and satiety. The system starts sending signals that you must stop eating when full. It also makes you eat when the stomach is empty. Everything has been perfectly timed and tuned.

However, obese people remain deprived of this automated system. They neither have any control over their satiety nor over their hunger.

Let us talk about the satiety hormone first.

Our body likes to store fat but this doesn't mean that it would want to keep hoarding unwanted fat too. Therefore, as soon as you start eating it begins releasing a hormone that signals your brain that the stores are being refilled. Soon when there is excess storage the hormones signal your body to stop eating. This condition is called satiety.

The hormone that signals this satiety is called 'Leptin'.

It is released by the fat stores. When you are in an unfed state the release of leptin is the lowest. As soon as you start eating it increases and it is the maximum when you are full. The high amount of leptin in your blood would mean that you don't need to eat anymore.

Understand Why Most Obese People Can't Resist Food

Unfortunately, this system malfunctions in the obese people and the cause of the malfunction are generally chronic inflammation in the fat cells. What happens afterward is the opposite.

When there is a chronic malfunction in your fat cells, they keep releasing leptin hormone at a moderate level all the time. The leptin is released by fat cells and the number of fat cells is higher in obese people, their body keep releasing high quantity of leptin hormone all the time. Either you are in a fed state of an empty stomach, there will always be the presence of leptin in your blood.

This should work as good because the presence of leptin would mean that you will feel satiated all the time and would eat less. This should happen in an ideal scenario but doesn't. High exposure to leptin hormone makes the receptive organ resistant to the leptin signals. This means that even though your body is releasing leptin in large quantities, you may never feel fully satisfied.

Ever wondered why some obese people like to eat so much. They may not have the hunger but they simply can't stop eating. It is not the temptation or love of food that causes the problem but leptin resistance.

This is a very serious problem as the body loses control over the fat-storage regulatory mechanism. Your body would keep releasing the leptin hormone at the same rate all the time. There would be no difference between the fed state and fasting state. Higher consumption of calories would again mean more storage and hence there comes no relief from obesity.

Another major reason for the development of leptin resistance is the high presence of free fatty acids in the bloodstream. These are also released by the fat cells and the higher the amount of fat deposit in the body, the greater would be the release of free fatty acids. They impair the ability of the brain to register the presence of leptin and hence you never really feel full.

Fasting and a good diet can give you a break from this vicious cycle. When you begin fasting for longer periods, the incessant release of leptin slows down. Generally, when people eat at frequent intervals, the leptin release keeps getting stimulated. However, when your body remains in a fasted state for longer than 20 hours, the leptin release also starts slowing down. Your brain can again experience the difference between the times when leptin release is high and the times when it is low and hence your satiety starts improving.

Inflammation of the fat cells is the root cause of the problem and that can also be tackled by eating anti-inflammatory foods. Food items rich in healthy fats and giving sugar, refined carbs and unhealthy fats a miss is always very helpful.

Longer fasting and anti-inflammatory food can help in restoring leptin sensitivity in your body. You would experience better control over your appetite. You would start feeling full after eating which doesn't happen in case of leptin resistance. In such cases, people simply keep eating but never feel full.

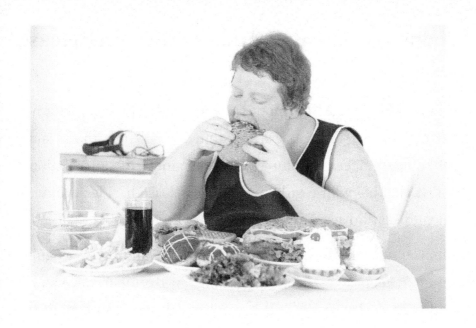

# Chapter 7: Normalization of Ghrelin Release

Ghrelin is the hunger hormone in your body. This is a hormone which performs several crucial functions other than simply stimulating hunger. Ghrelin release promotes the production of HGH. It also helps in regulating insulin release besides promoting the healthy cardiovascular system.

Normalize ghrelin levels can also help in improved cognitive function. People especially battling with neurodegenerative disorders like Alzheimers and Parkinson's disease can benefit a lot by normalized ghrelin levels.

Ghrelin release is highest when you are hungry and lowest when you are full. High ghrelin levels do promote HGH production but that only occurs when you are in a fasted state and insulin levels are low. If you are eating frequent meals and your ghrelin levels remain high, it can have adverse effects on your health. The high concentration of ghrelin in such cases will lead to overeating and you would accumulate more fat.

Foods with high added sugar content are bad for you. They do not suppress your ghrelin levels and keep getting added as fat. This increases the risk of obesity.

Intermittent fasting can help you in taking full advantage of normalized ghrelin levels. When you are observing extended periods of fast your ghrelin levels increase and they facilitate the production of HGH. This hormone helps in burning fat and promotes muscle growth. The more exercise you do in the fasted state the better the results would be.

Longer periods of ghrelin release also promote cognitive function. You feel sharper and more alert.

Therefore, to get the best advantage of high ghrelin levels it is important to remain in the fasted state.

Your ghrelin levels are at their peak when you are hungry and go down after you have consumed your meals. Eating frequently and having foods rich in sugar cause cravings and do not lower the ghrelin levels. You remain hungry and overeat as a result. This leads to obesity.

So, the ghrelin hormone acts as a double-edged sword. It can work to promote good health if you observe intermittent fasting but will lead to fat accumulation if you keep overeating.

Frequently eating food products rich in added sugar can also lead to adverse effects. Your ghrelin levels wouldn't go down even after eating and your hunger also wouldn't subside.

Ghrelin function is inverse to the leptin function. When your ghrelin levels go down your leptin release increases and you feel satisfied. However, if your ghrelin levels remain high, you wouldn't feel satisfied and keep feeling the urge to eat more. It will lead to weight gain.

Intermittent fasting can help you in avoiding this problem. It will normalize your ghrelin levels and let you have the complete advantage of high ghrelin release.

It is one of the reasons that exercise is always the best on an empty stomach. While you are a bit hungry your HGH production is high and you are able to exercise better and get the best fat cutting advantages.

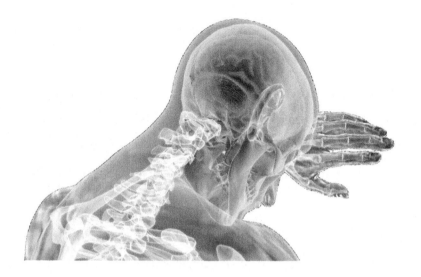

# Chapter 8: Lowers the Risk of Chronic Inflammations

Most of the problems that occur in our body may look like the result of some particular incident but they aren't. All long term disorders that our body develops are the result of chronic inflammations.

Inflammation in itself is not a particularly bad thing. In fact, it is the safety mechanism of your body to repair itself. However, the problem begins when the repair work starts once but never really ends. Such a condition is called chronic inflammation.

For instance, diabetes may look like a problem related to poor sugar control. One day you realize that your body is not able to manage the sugar levels properly anymore. For you, the problem began that day. However, the problem may have started years ago at the least for your body. The tolerance level of our body is very high but everything has its limits.

Chronic inflammation of all kinds is bad. It can cause health issues like heart diseases, hypertension, thyroid issues, obesity, chronic pain, diabetes, migraines, and even cancer. Not only this, autoimmune diseases like ulcerative colitis, rheumatoid arthritis, multiple sclerosis, and Crohn's disease are also caused by chronic inflammation.

You may be at a higher risk of falling prey to chronic inflammation if:

- You are obese or overweight
- Your diet is unhealthy
- You don't do much physical activity
- You have too much stress in your life

Fasting for longer hours can help you in dealing with these problems. It brings down the oxidative stress in your body. Oxidative stress is a big reason for chronic inflammations to begin and spread.

It also lowers the presence of free fatty acids in your blood. The levels of LDL, triglycerides, and bad cholesterol also go down in your body.

Fasting also helps in lowering the levels of C-reactive protein in your blood. A high presence of C-reactive protein increases the risk of inflammations.

These are the factors that cause chronic inflammations and fasting helps to lower the presence of all these factors.

Besides other things, the biggest victim of chronic inflammations is your brain. Chronic inflammation affects the levels of Brain-derived neurotrophic factor (BDNF). If the levels of BDNF are low, the neuroplasticity in the brain cells will go down. What this means is that your brain cells have an amazing ability to regenerate at a high pace, this power is called neuroplasticity. However, lower BDNF levels impair this ability and then cognitive functions start getting affected. Lower neuroplasticity can also lead to shrinkage of the brain in size. This also leads to the development of neurodegenerative disorders like Alzheimer's and Parkinson 's disease.

Fasting can help in increasing the levels of BDNF. Neuroplasticity also increases and your brain cells are able to regenerate at a normal rate.

Fasting also helps in curing chronic inflammations in other regions like your blood sugar levels, insulin resistance, fat accumulation, etc.

It is a great way to treat the problems concerning your liver diseases. Being the only organ in the body to have regenerative ability, the liver is an amazing organ. It can treat most of the problems it faces. However, our current lifestyle and poor eating habits put a lot of stress on the liver. They can lead to inflammation and you may face problems like fatty liver disease. Fasting has a very remedial impact on this condition.

The best thing to counter inflammation that fasting does is that it lowers the oxidative stress in your body. The oxidative stress is the prime cause of most of the problems. When free radicals increase in the blood a lot, they cause oxidative stress. Fasting helps in the utilization of these free radicals for producing energy and hence the oxidative goes down.

So, if you want to stay healthy and fit, fasting can help you in a big way.

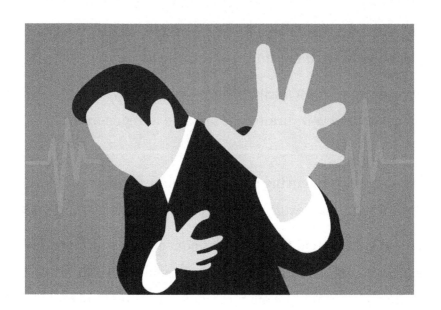

# Chapter 9: Lowers the Risk of Heart Diseases

You can hear cholesterol in every other food commercial these days. The food production industry has brandished cholesterol as the main villain. However, it is not the whole truth.

Cholesterol is made from the fat in your body and it is essential for the production of various hormones, especially the ones required for making you virile and fertile. It has several other functions like it is used by your body as a Band-Aid. Whenever there is an injury to your heart vessels, cholesterol deposits are used to mend the damage.

The biggest heart problem people face is blockage of vessels and there are high cholesterol deposits. So, people conveniently blame cholesterol for the problem. If cholesterol deposits wouldn't have mended the damaged blood vessels, you may not have survived even this long. The real problem is caused by the Ischemic injuries your heart faces from time to time. Chronic inflammation, stressful life, and unhealthy foods are the primary cause of the problem and not the cholesterol.

Every time cholesterol mends the vessels, the arteries get narrow. Chronic inflammation even accelerates the process. If unchecked, this would cause atherosclerosis, a condition in which the cholesterol and fatty-rich plaque deposits restrict the blood vessels.

If you really want to lower the risk of heart diseases, it is important to root out the cause of the problem and that is chronic inflammation, stress, and poor food choice. Diabetes, high blood pressure, and a sedentary lifestyle also contribute hugely to the problem.

People even blame high levels of triglycerides for heart problems. Like cholesterol, they also have an indirect role to play in the problem. However, they are also not bad. Your body can use triglycerides for producing energy. The levels of triglycerides depend upon the kind of food you consume. Sugar-rich food would lead to higher production of triglycerides.

Fasting can help you in lowering your bad cholesterol and triglyceride levels. When your body goes into ketosis, it uses free fatty acids as the main fuel. The liver releases ketones that can metabolize the free fatty acids and triglycerides for producing energy and hence the risk of heart disease would be less.

However, it is important to note that high-cholesterol level is not the sole reason for heart disease and neither a true indicator of heart problems.

People have a great fear that if they eat high-fat food, they may face heart problems. This is not true. The reason for the high buildup of LDL or bad cholesterol in your body is insulin resistance and not high-fat food. In fact, almost 80% of cholesterol present in your body is produced in your liver itself. The percentage of dietary cholesterol is only 20% and it has no role in play in the health of your heart.

If you want to ensure good heart health, then your focus must be on lowering insulin resistance in your body and increasing physical activity. Fasting helps you in decreasing insulin resistance. If you also start doing exercise, the risk of heart problems would also go down. Exercises put your body under mind positive stress. They also help in the release of nitric oxide. It makes your blood vessels expand a bit and hence their ability to absorb Ischemic injuries improves.

You can ensure better heart health with One Meal a Day fasting as it has a very high impact on insulin resistance. Your body becomes sensitive to insulin and hence the blood sugar levels in your body remain in control. If the blood sugar levels remain high for long consistently, it will cause blood vessels hardening and this will go to increase the risk of damage.

Fasting also lowers the amount of visceral fat in your body. This is the harmful fat surrounding your vital organs. It dumps a lot of free fatty acids in the blood that cause inflammation. The lower the amount of visceral fat the better the heart health would be.

It is a proven fact that fasting has a very positive role in lowering blood pressure. Fasting decreases your salt intake and increases the intake of water. As the insulin sensitivity in your body improves, the blood pressure also starts to go down. So, you will become less prone to injuries caused by the heart by high blood pressure.

Fasting is an easy and effective way to ensure good heart health. You can bring a big change in your health by simply showing some control over your eating habits.

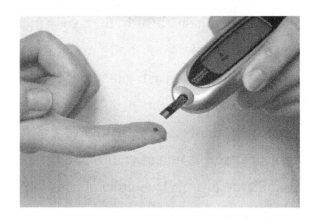

# Chapter 10: Helps in Diabetes

Diabetes has emerged as one of the biggest killers in the world. In the US alone, there are more than 110 million people who are either suffering from diabetes or prediabetes. Although no disease can be characterized as good this one, in particular, is the evilest one.

Diabetes makes you a slave of medicines. It is a disease for which medical science has no cure yet and all the doctors can do is manage the blood sugar levels to keep you running. Poor management of blood sugar levels can lead to severe complications and even multiple organ failure. High sugar levels also harden the arteries reducing the functionality of the vital organs.

Fasting is the only way to ease this problem a bit. It helps in the development of insulin sensitivity and your body can get better control over blood sugar management. However, if you are already suffering from diabetes, you must consult your doctor and undergo regular tests to ensure that there are no erratic changes in the blood sugar levels.

Fasting can help you with diabetes in the following ways:

Helps in Decreasing Insulin Resistance

Insulin resistance is one of the major reasons for developing prediabetes which then matures to diabetes. If your body becomes more insulin sensitive, this problem can be avoided. Your body will be able to absorb blood sugar faster and there wouldn't be a problem of high blood sugar levels for longer periods. It also helps the pancreas by lowering the pressure on it to keep pumping insulin.

Helps in Weight Loss

Excess weight increases the problems in diabetes. You would be able to have much better control over diabetes if your weight remains under check. Fasting is a sure-shot method of bringing weight under control.

# Gives a Boost to Metabolism

High metabolism plays a key role in managing diabetes successfully. Fasting is a good way to boost metabolism. There are several studies that have proven that you can give a great boost to your metabolism through fasting.

So, if you are suffering from diabetes, you must start practicing fasting. You must also keep your doctor in the loop as managing the blood sugar levels, in the beginning, can get tricky and the doctor might have to adjust your medications at regular intervals. However, it is a way through which you can bring a substantial change in your condition.

# Chapter 11: Promotes Anti-aging

We all want to stay young and healthy. However, age has its effect on all of us and we age. As long as we are aging at the right speed things should be good. However, the current trend shows that people are showing signs of early aging. Stressful life, environmental factors, pollution, and chronic inflammations have a deep impact on our health. They make us age prematurely. This is a problem that needs to be tackled.

Most people consider premature aging to be a cosmetic problem. However, it simply isn't that. If your body is showing signs of aging it means that is something very wrong going on inside that needs your immediate attention.

There are 3 main factors responsible for early aging:

1. Oxidative Stress
2. High Free-Radical Damage
3. Low Glycosaminoglycans (GAG) levels

Free radicals and oxidative stress are interconnected as the higher the levels of free radicals are in your body, the higher oxidative stress would be. This would also cause chronic inflammations. We have already discussed that free radical damage can be reduced by the following fasting. It helps in lowering the levels of visceral fat in the body which is the main source of dumping free radicals. It also helps in reducing oxidative stress. Your body gets into a better position to fight chronic inflammations that may bring early signs of aging.

The main sign of early aging is brought by a slower rate of formation of collagen in the body. It is a structural protein found in skin and connective tissues. GAG is the main chemical that keeps the collagen hydrated and your skin doesn't get wrinkles. It also repairs the damage caused to the collagen. The GAG levels go down in your body when the liver stops functioning properly. Fasting can help in reviving the production of GAG and you wouldn't have to face early signs of aging.

The chief hormone responsible for bringing this positive change is Insulin-Like Growth Factor Number 1 (IGF-1). If your body starts producing IGF-1 in healthy quantities, signs of aging can be reversed.

Some Important Ways to Boost the Production of IGF-1

# Lower Insulin Levels

High insulin levels in the blood stop the production of IGF-1 in your liver. Your liver would only be able to produce IGF-1 if the insulin levels remain low. This can be made possible through fasting as we know that fasting has a very important role in keeping the insulin levels under check.

# Better Sleep and Cortisol Levels

The production of IGF-1 is higher when you are asleep. Because it is a repair hormone, its production is generally at its peak during your sleep. You can boost production by sleeping for optimum hours. The same goes for stress. The higher the levels of stress hormone in your blood the lower will be the production of other hormones as it puts the body in an energy conservation mode. Leading a healthy and positive lifestyle can boost the production of IGF-1 and lower the stress hormone.

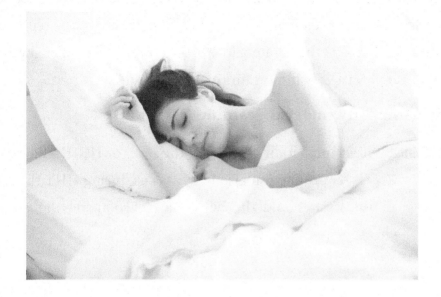

## Improve the Health of Your Liver

The liver is the place where the production of IGF-1 takes place. If your liver is healthy and functioning well it will be in a better position to produce IGF-1. Fasting has a very positive impact on the health of your liver. You can also improve the health of your liver by reducing the intake of toxins through healthy food. Lower intake of sugar and carbs also plays a very important role in the process.

## High-Intensity Interval Training (HIIT)

HIIT has a great impact on increasing the level of HGH. The same goes for IGF-1. Its production also increases as during HIIT there is damage to the tissues and the body starts producing the repair hormone in large quantities.

# Chapter 12: Autophagy

Autophagy is an amazing process. It is a marvel that our body has. It remained unknown to humankind for centuries and has been studied in detail in recent years. A Japanese scientist by the name of Yoshinori Oshumi did a detailed study on the concept and found that our body has the inherent ability to treat most of its problems and the process through which it does that is known as Autophagy.

Most of the problems in the body are caused due to the accumulation of waste, toxins, and parasites. The body becomes inefficient in its functioning and several processes start self-harming. As long as the body remains in an energy surplus mode, it never feels the need to make the processes efficient as there is no need for conservation of something that's present in abundance. However, as soon as there would be a severe energy deficit, the body would begin purging the inefficient process and that mechanism is known as autophagy.

Our body has trillions of cells and there are even a greater number of germs that live inside our body. Some of these germs have a positive impact but there are many that are simply parasites feeding on the energy produced by the body. Pathogens like fungi, molds, and bacteria come under this category.

When you begin fasting and your body senses that no energy supply is coming from outside, it feels the need to start autophagy. This process starts selective purging and roots out all the pathogens that are not playing any beneficial role in the body.

Our body produces millions of new cells every day. The process is unending and fast. In the process of producing new cells, there are some cells that are not produced well. They have structural issues and they play no active part in the body. When the body goes into autophagy, it identifies all such cells and starts recycling them for producing new cells and also releases energy from them. This means that the body would start using up all the useless things in the body for producing energy. You will not only get new cells but the waste in the body would also get cleaned. These cells take up space and cause clutter. They may also cause problems in the body.

A part of the same process also involves stopping the growth of unwanted cells. Cancer is also a disease in which there is an uncontrolled and unregulated growth of some cells. When your body goes into autophagy it also identifies these cells and stops their growth. There are studies still going on in this direction but scientists believe that autophagy can play a very important role in stopping the growth of cancer in the body.

Treating cancer through other methods in a reliable way is very difficult as the cancer cells are also similar to your body cells. The medicines that kill the cancer cells also kill normal cells. These cells behave in a normal way and have the regrowth also in the same way. The only difference between the cancer cells and normal cells is that the normal cells can function both on energy produced through glucose or fat whereas the cancer cells can only use the energy produced through glucose. When your body goes through autophagy the supply of glucose fuel stops completely. The ketosis begins and the cells start using the energy produced from fat as fuel. However, the cancer cells are unable to do that and they start shrinking.

Autophagy begins a catabolic process in which it starts purging all the cells in the body that are not playing an active role. It is a process through which the body becomes very energy efficient.

# How to Begin Autophagy

Autophagy is an automatic process that would begin when you stop supplying energy from outside. It means that you would need to do fasting. Generally, it is believed that the body enters into autophagy after 36 hours of fasting as it starts feeling the need to conserve energy for the longer possibility of survival. However, once autophagy begins, even shorter fasts longer than 20 hours can give you the benefits of autophagy. Dr. Yoshinori Oshumi received the Nobel Peace prize of 2016 for his work on autophagy and further studies are underway to understand the benefits we can get from the process.

Autophagy has 2 main benefits:

# Cleaning of the Body

This process starts purging anything and everything that's unwanted in the body. It is a very important process as it makes your body more efficient. It helps in strengthening the immune system and make the body more resistant to diseases.

# Stops the Progression of Diseases

There are several useless processes going on in the body like chronic inflammations that are not contributing anything and using up energy. Autophagy stops all such processes and brings you in a better position to fight diseases.

If done properly, you can lose a lot of weight through the process and also get healthier. Autophagy is a complete wellness concept in itself and can take you a long way towards good health.

# Part III

# Chapter 13: Understanding One Meal A Day Routine

One Meal a Day routine as the name suggests simply involves eating once a day. It is a form of intermittent fasting. Therefore, to understand One Meal a Day routine it is important for you to have a general overview of Intermittent Fasting.

Intermittent Fasting

Intermittent fasting is a very simple method of bringing variation in your eating patterns. It involves longer fasting windows and shorter eating windows within a day. It isn't complete fasting as you would be allowed to eat. However, it has a lot of health benefits as it helps in lowering the health risks and increasing your body's ability to lose weight faster and fight diseases better.

There are several popular intermittent fasting routines that are followed all over the world. The most commonly followed routine is 16:8. This routine involves observing a fasting window of 16 hours in a day and eating within the 8 hours window.

The next routine is the 20:4 routine or the warrior diet. It requires you to fast for 20 hours and have one or two meals within the 4-hour eating window.

Next comes, the One Meal a Day routine that involves fasting for 23 hours a day and eating a single meal within a one hours eating window.

There are other intermittent fasting routines like alternate day fasting routine that involves fasting for complete 24 hours and then eating normally the next day. This routine needs to be followed throughout the week.

There are also longer fasting routine involving fasting for longer periods up to 36 hours. These fasts can be observed once a month and they are very helpful in detoxification and cleansing of the body. They also help in kick-starting the process of autophagy.

## Important Thing to Note

Intermittent fasting in general and One Meal a Day routine, in particular, isn't a diet. The weight loss industry has engraved the idea of the diet with all efforts to lose weight. One Meal a Day is a routine. There are no elaborate rules to follow. There are no calories to count. There is no watch to be kept on what you can or can't eat. There will be no guilt conscious after every meal you have.

Intermittent fasting is a way of life. It is a lifestyle change that you will have to incorporate into your life. It isn't something that can happen overnight. You must incorporate this life change into your life slowly and give it the due time. The results will be phenomenal as the weight that goes away wouldn't come back. There will be no fear of weight relapse as your body would become capable of losing and maintaining that weight.

# One Meal A Day Routine

There is no doubt that for anyone beginning intermittent fasting this routine can look scary and difficult. We have a very deep relationship with food. It is not only related to our physical needs but also has a psychological impact. However, if a person is facing a problem like obesity then there is already an excess of stored energy that needs to be spent first. By showing some self-control and discipline one can easily follow this routine and get all the health benefits discussed earlier in the book.

Any kind of fasting requires self-control and discipline. To most people 16:8 may look like a very easy routine. However, when you begin it, the process is equally difficult. You would need to train your body and mind to remain in the fasted state for that period. The same goes for one meal a day. It may look like a long and difficult routine but you don't have to begin with it. You must always begin with shorter routines and gradually move on to one meal a day and then it would be similar to all the other routines.

## Hunger Is As Much Psychological Phenomenon As It Is Physiological

The biggest worry people have while beginning any kind of fasting is that they wouldn't be able to bear hunger. However, it is important to understand that hunger doesn't always indicate your body's need to eat. It is mostly your desire to have food that your body doesn't require. In fact, if you are battling weight issues, it means that your body has ample energy reserves to run the body efficiently. Going without food for a much longer period wouldn't harm you at all. Yet, the more weight you carry the more inclined you feel to eat.

This temptation of food is not a result of your body's need to eat but caused by inflammation in the fat cells and food cravings. Both these issues can be handled easily by practicing fasting regularly and slowly increasing the fasting time.

Psychological hunger is usually very sudden and forces you to have food. The physiological hunger develops slowly and it gets regulated with time. The release of ghrelin hormone that regulates hunger gets automatically timed as per your eating schedule. It means that if you are following a certain gap between meals you are least likely to experience physical hunger before your scheduled eating time.

So, if you are concerned that you will not be able to remain in the fasted state for very long, your fears are unfounded. With a little practice and self-control, anyone can switch to One Meal a Day routine and get all the health benefits.

One Meal a Day routine is very simple to follow and has the least complexities. You get one meal a day and in that meal, you can eat up to your satisfaction.

There are four simple rules to follow:

# 1 Hour

You will get one hour a day to have your meal. This can be the most satisfying one hour of your day. You would have been in the fasted state for 23 hours and the hunger would be at its peak. Your gut would be ready to process the meal quickly as it would have easily processed your last meal by then. This is the best arrangement for your vital processes as well as your gut.

In this 1 hour, you can enjoy your meal up to your heart's content without worrying about the number of calories you are consuming. Remember, intermittent fasting routines lay great emphasis on 'when' rather than 'what' or 'how much'. This means that while having this meal you would have no guilt of having food despite being overweight.

# 1 Meal

You will only get one meal a day. This single meal of your day should provide you all the nutrients, vitamins, and minerals. You will not be able to consume any other meal for the next 23 hours and therefore this meal should be very balanced and nutritious. You must choose the right kind of things in this meal that can provide you the required nutrition.

The ideal ratio of the content of your meals should be:

Fat: 70-75%

Protein: 20-25%

Carbohydrates: 5-10%

If your meal has this composition, you will be able to get all the nutrients without overstuffing yourself or feeling bloated.

The fat is compact and provides more calories as compared to protein and carbs.

The protein is also compact and helps you feel satisfied for longer without food.

You must consume fresh green leafy vegetables and whole grains to get your carbs. The green leafy vegetables are full of antioxidants, vitamins, and minerals. They also have a lot of fiber but add very few calories to your system. You can eat them as much as you want and they would keep your gut busy for longer. You must avoid refined carbs and sugar in your meals as they will not only cause cravings but will also load empty calories into your system. You would start feeling food cravings faster and the hunger would become unmanageable.

## 1 Plate

Keeping the quantity of food in mind is also very important. Eating after 23 hours can tempt you into thinking that eating more would help in remaining in the fasted state for longer. This is not correct. Overeating will only complicate things for you. If you eat too much you may feel bloated or overstuffed and that would cause discomfort. You must make it a rule to not eat more than one standard plate. It would obviously have more food than a regular meal but help you in preventing overeating. The better your balance of the macronutrients is the lesser would be the food in your plate. You should get around

1800 calories from this meal. This will ensure that your calorie intake remains in check and your body gets a chance to burn more.

## 1 Beverage

There are certain permitted beverages that you can consume even in your fasting period. Unsweetened black tea or coffee, fresh lime, and water are some of the things that wouldn't add calories to your system and hence you can have them in your fasting period too. However, in this eating window, you can have one beverage of your choice. It can be anything that you like but it is always wise not to consume beverages with very high sugar content.

If you can follow these four simple rules in your life, One Meal a Day routine will have no complexities for you.

# Chapter 14: Preparation- Understanding the Difficult Part and Dealing with It

Weight loss measures of all kinds are difficult yet people follow them. However, we see that most people are never able to reap the full benefit of the measures. It is not the complete failure of the process or the practitioner but the difficulty of maintaining the routine that poses the real problem.

We all know that if we do rigorous exercise, we will burn calories. Our calorie expenditure will increase and if we are able to lower the intake there has to be some degree of fat burn. Yet, People with consistent gym memberships fail to get into shape. The same is the story of diets.

Diets are the most painful. They are restrictive and have a profound impact on physique as well as the mind of the practitioner. Yet, you can see hundreds of people who have been on some kind of diet but haven't brought any significant change in their life.

People even take the extreme route of surgical intervention for weight loss. Bariatric surgeries are a norm these days. People get under the knife and have their guts altered surgically to bring a change in their diets. Procedures like gastric banding, gastric sleeve, or gastric bypass ensure that the body helps you in restricting your food intake. However, even the people who have been through these procedures experience weight relapse.

The most difficult part of weight loss is to follow a lifestyle that helps you in losing and maintaining that weight. People generally give their complete attention to the regimen but pay very little attention to their lifestyle. They follow diets religiously irrespective of the severity of the routine. However, every diet comes with an end date. As soon as they get off the diet they feel free to eat whatever they like and in whatever quantity they wish. Although they might have got off the diet, the body is always in the fat- storage mode. Hence, weight relapse is even faster.

The same goes for fitness routines. People start with the toughest routines they can pick. They work very hard. They pump iron for hours in the gym and even start experiencing results. However, it is impractical for most of us to pump iron in gyms for hours on a regular basis. Soon the reality kicks in that rigorous fitness routines are tough, excruciating, time taking, and exhausting. While we all want to lose weight we also need to have our day jobs to run our livelihood. Soon, the realization draws upon people and the time devoted to fitness routines starts to go down. People even start skipping the gym. However, when people start the gym they also get on a specific diet to supplement your routine. Although they start reducing the time devoted to the gym, they pay little attention to the diet they had increased. The results are horrific.

The real problem is not that these weight loss measures don't work. The real problem is that they aren't lifelong options. It is very difficult to maintain difficult routines for very long. On the contrary, the body is always in the fat-storage mode. It likes to store more and fatter as that is the best strategy from the survival point of view. This is the prime bone of contention.

Consistency in Weight Loss Strategy

If you want your weight loss strategy to work, consistency is the word for you. You can't pick one style for yourself and drop it at your convenience. Your weight loss strategy has to be a part of your lifestyle.

## **Slow and Steady Transition**

Another problem with most weight loss strategies is that people begin with the most difficult routines as they want fast results. There has to be a difference between weight loss and instant noodles. The tummy tires didn't develop overnight. Trying to get rid of them instantly is a poor strategy. The results would be horrific and you would be sending shock signals to your body.

Imagine you had a pretty sedentary lifestyle and then one-day realization draws upon you that you are fat and you get on a rampage to shed the weight. From a sedentary lifestyle to pumping iron in the gym for one hour twice a day will be a complete shock for your body. The first reaction of your body would be a revolt. From muscle cramps and fatigue to dizziness, the symptoms can vary. However, one thing is for sure, your body is not going to appreciate it.

If you want any weight loss strategy to work for you, it has to be slow and steady so that your body can adjust to the positive change.

# How to Incorporate 'One Meal A Day'

The best strategy is to go slow and steady as stated above. If you believe that staying hungry for a whole day would be a welcome change for your body, think again. It is neither correct nor advisable. There are several steps in-between that you will have to take. You will have to be consistent and move slowly.

Your body doesn't look at the food in the same way as you see it while you are on a diet. It is a reason diets are so much detested. You will have to get your body to develop the ability to stay without food. It can only be done in a systematic way. Given below are the ways through which you can reach a One Meal A Day milestone with ease and stay on it comfortably. However, it is important for you to understand that you won't get there tomorrow. It can take months at least before your body gets ready to remain without food for that long without food on a daily basis.

- Every step of the way needs to be followed with consistency.
- You must stay at every level for a fortnight at least even after you have started feeling comfortable.
- You MUST NOT bypass any step.
- You must only move forward to the next step only when your body starts feeling fully adjusted to the routine.

# First Step - Eliminate Snacks from Your Daily Routine

Snacks are the prime reasons our body is never really able to relax and constantly remains in the food processing mode. Snacks are highly responsible for the rising levels of insulin resistance. They keep your gut engaged and also confuse your system.

If you are overweight or obese, it means that you are in an energy surplus mode. However, snacks never really let your body rest. They are the prime reason behind blood sugar spikes in your body.

The first thing you must do is eliminate all kinds of snacks from your routine. This also includes all the sweetened beverages and tit-bits that may add calories to your system. You must limit yourself to 3 meals a day and believe me, even they are unnecessary.

The best way to do this is to have a balanced diet. Any meal with a proper quantity of macronutrients like fat, protein, and carbs can help you in going from one meal to another without feeling the urge to have snacks.

The cravings that you may still feel are only a result of psychological hunger. Staying away from sugar, refined flours, and processed food that is highly laced with sugar and preservative will help you in doing so.

Try to eat food items that can keep your gut engaged for long in a positive way. Eating fiber-rich food items is a great way to do so. Such foods take a lot of time to get digested and hence you wouldn't feel unwanted food cravings.

You must adjust your body to this routine where you only have 3 meals a day at fixed intervals. You must learn to avoid all temptations of food in-between your meals. Once you get used to this routine, follow it at least for a fortnight before moving ahead.

## Second Step- Having All Your Meals within 12-Hour Span

This one should be easy once you have eliminated snacks from your routine. It is very easy for us to remain in the fasted state for 8-10 hours. This is the time when we are sleeping. Make it a rule to eat anything a few hours after the sun comes up and have to your last meal of the day before the sun goes down. This isn't very difficult once you have started exercising a little bit of self-control.

It can be difficult for you if your diet has a lot of sugar in it. Sugar or carbohydrate-rich diet loads your system with empty calories. While you are eating you start feeling fuller very fast as your system gets flooded with calories. However, this satiety wouldn't last long as although your bloodstream gets loaded with calories, your gut doesn't get much to digest. This confuses your body and the hunger pangs start developing very soon. That's why some people find it very difficult to keep their hands off the food. Such people start feeling hungry soon after dinner and may not find it unusual to raid the kitchen in the middle of the night.

The solution to this problem is also the right mix of the macronutrients. The more fat and protein-rich diet you have, the longer you would be able to keep off your hunger pangs.

You must follow even this routine for at least a fortnight and only move ahead when you experience that the need to have food outside the eating window has gone away.

Third Step- Extend the Fasting Period to 16 Hours

This would be the beginning of the actual fat loss routine. 16 hours of fasting window can have a profound impact on your insulin resistance and it will help in developing insulin sensitivity.

Observing a fasting window of at least 16 hours a day will help your body experience positive stress. This is also very important for developing the ability to fight chronic illnesses.

Till this stage, nothing much would have changed. Only fasting hours increase from 12-16. You will still be able to enjoy 3 meals a day within the 8 hours eating window. There will not be any kind of food restrictions and you can freely eat anything you deem fit, as long as it is healthy. However, this is the time you must start observing restraint in your food choices and the number of meals consumed. Although you can have 3 meals a day, the 8-hour eating window doesn't leave enough room for distributing 3 meals if you are consuming a balanced diet.

You should ideally be having a heavy meal at the beginning of the day as you will be entering the active phase of your day. By the time you begin feeling the hunger pangs, you would be near the time for your last meal. If you experience hunger within the day, you must not have something very heavy as it would make you feel lethargic. Try to have some salad or fruit to suppress your hunger.

The last meal of the day should be comparatively light as you would not be working much as having something heavy can make you feel bloated or uncomfortable.

This way, you will be able to perfect the 16:8 intermittent fasting routine without experiencing any great difficulty. Having a balanced diet is critical as it will help you in going from one meal to another without feeling the need to have snacks.

16 hours can look like a long time to remain in a fasted state but in reality, it isn't much if you plan properly. The best way to carry it out is to have the last meal of the day as early as possible. Generally, the last phase of the fast is more difficult as the hunger pangs get intense. However, if you begin the fasting early in the evening, you can pass most of this time in your sleep. If you are a night person you can time your beginning of the fast a bit late as you would be getting up late in the morning.

In any case, it is important that you have the last meal of the day at least 3-4 hours before going to bed. This facilitates proper digestion of food and hence the levels of insulin go down faster. It also helps in higher production of HGH which also aids your weight loss efforts. The load on your digestion system also goes down.

You should also start shifting the first meal of your day to later so that instead of having breakfast and lunch you can have brunch. This will again help in burning fat faster. The longer you remain in the fasted state the more your body would be bound to metabolize the fat in your body as it will not be getting energy from external sources.

# Step Four- 20-Hour Fasting

Things start to get tough here and you should not move to this step until you have become very comfortable with the 16 hours fasting. Once you are able to successfully shift your breakfast without any noticeable discomfort you will know that you are ready to move to the next step.

The 20-hour fasting is not very different from 16-hour fasting it only has the element of 4 extended hours of fasting. However, this may not be as easy as 16-hour fasting. This is difficult to master routine. You will most definitely experience hunger pangs as they are inevitable. However, the extended fasting hours and the hunger pangs aid the production of hormones that lead to fat burning.

At this stage, it will be very important for you to start consuming a highly balanced and nutritious diet. You get only 4 hours eating window within a day. You can spread a single meal within this four-hour eating window or have two meals, the choice will be yours.

The best strategy is to have something light like fruits and salads at the beginning of the fast and have a complete meal at the end. If you start with a heavy meal, you may not be able to eat much within four hours.

This is the routine you must follow the longest before moving on to One Meal A Day routine.

# Step Five- 23-Hour Fasting or One Meal A Day

Like all other fasting routines, this one is also similar to the previous ones in nature. You will need to remain in the fasted state for 23 hours and have a complete meal in the 1-hour eating window.

Hunger pangs will be severe and stronger and there is no getting around them. We have got so much used to the routine of eating several meals a day that this routine may take much longer to perfect.

The only thing that can help you the most is a highly balanced diet. You must remember that most people with any kind of appetite will not be able to eat much in a single meal. Yet, you will have to consume 1500-1800 calories and get all the vitamins, minerals, and fiber from it. Proper distribution of the macronutrients is essential.

The fat content in your food must be 70-75%. You should include healthy fats like nuts, seeds, fish, cheese, eggs, etc. to get all the required fat.

The protein is required by the body and it must make 20-25% of your food. Protein is slow to digest and helps you in feeling fuller for longer.

The ratio of carbs should be the least as they release energy quickly and make you crave for food faster. However, carbs are also important as you get vitamins, minerals, antioxidants, phytonutrients, trace minerals, and fiber from them. You must include a lot of green leafy vegetables in your meal. You can eat them as much as you want without counting calories as they add very few calories to your system. But, they are full of other important nutrients. They also have a lot of fiber that will keep your gut engaged.

One Meal a Day routine is a lifestyle change that you will have to incorporate. This means that you must not take the liberties of cheat days. This routine doesn't prohibit eating or drinking anything during the eating window. Hence, there will not be a temptation to eat.

It is an ideal routine if you want to lose weight, burn fat, and stay healthy.

One Meal a Day may look like a rigorous and difficult to follow a routine but it isn't if you give your body the right conditioning and transition time. It is important to remember that obesity is a chronic problem. The fat accumulation in your body hasn't happened in a day and your body likes to accumulate fat. Dealing with that fat cannot be very quick. The quick weight loss methods are unreliable and the results are very inconsistent and temporary. The weight relapses faster than it went away and you would be standing back to square one in no time if you follow the quick fixes.

The best way to deal with the issue of obesity is to give your body the time to heal itself and counter the factors that lead to obesity. It is very important to understand that obesity is a result of the health issues your body has been facing, it isn't the cause. The causes of obesity are insulin resistance, diabetes, metabolic disorders, and other such problems. If you want to fight obesity then the fight has to be against all these issues and the problem would get resolved on its own. Once your body gets the right conditions, it will be able to burn the fat and utilize it for producing energy. You wouldn't need to undertake costly fad diets, overprices gym memberships or medical help.

Sticking to the routine is the most important thing if you want to get rid of the excess weight and burn fat to stay healthy and fit.

# Chapter 15: Things to Expect

## The Bad

There is no denying the fact that fasting for 23 hours a day isn't an easy task. There will be times in the beginning when you may start feeling frustrated. However, if you feel so there is no reason to be alarmed as it is common to feel so even on calorie restrictive diets too. Symptoms of physical discomfort like headache, nausea, and weakness are also common. The good thing is that all these symptoms are temporary and would go away very soon. If you make the transition to 23-hour fasting slowly these symptoms may not arise at all while following One Meal a Day routine. You would experience them early on and your body would get well adjusted to them by the time you get into the serious routine.

Still, there are some common symptoms that may appear at several stages. This chapter will help you in understanding the problems you may face and the ways to deal with them easily. If you are experiencing these symptoms then there is no reason to worry, in fact, you should feel happy that your body has started to adjust to the routine and it would soon start burning fat.

## Hunger Pangs

Hunger pangs are very common and even if you make the transition slowly as per the advice, you may still feel the hunger pangs troubling you. Hunger is a very important phenomenon. It is the push your body gives you to keep working towards bringing food. It is the motivation behind all the progress humankind has made throughout history. It is very natural for the gut to release ghrelin once the food in the gut gets digested. The hunger pangs are a signal to your brain to motivate you to eat. However, it is a mechanical process and every time you feel hungry doesn't mean that you necessarily need to eat.

Your gut releases ghrelin as per the schedule and it is mostly associated with the usual time of your eating. It means that if you are habitual of eating after you finish brushing your teeth in the morning, you will feel hunger irrespective of the fact that you ate a few hours ago. It is less about hunger and more about timing. However, the ghrelin release is always in spurts. It means, the gut would start releasing ghrelin at mealtime but would stop the release of the hormone after a while if you don't eat anything. It is a reason the hunger pangs are stronger for a while but subside later even if you don't eat anything.

The best way to avoid hunger pangs and the distress they cause is to keep yourself occupied. If you are sitting idle when you feel the hunger pangs the temptation to eat would get stronger. Your mind wouldn't stop thinking about food no matter how much you try. Keep yourself very busy in the last leg of your fasting schedule as the hunger pangs would be stronger and very real in this period.

Drinking non-caloric beverages like unsweetened black tea or coffee can also help in dealing with hunger pangs. These beverages suppress your hunger very much. You can also drink fresh lime water or plain water to push your hunger strongly. It will also help you in remaining hydrated.

## Cravings

Cravings are nothing unusual. Most of us have cravings for food items especially the ones that are sweet or spicy as mostly these things are loaded with calories and carbs. If your food has a lot of sugar you will find dealing with cravings all the more difficult. The best way out is to stay away from refined sugar. The processed food that we get in the superstores is loaded with sugar. All the fat-free food heavily publicized in the market is also loaded with sugar as taking out fat from the food also takes away its taste. Hence, sugar is added to make it palatable. Reading the labels carefully before purchasing the food items is very important. Food items that have sugar, fructose, and syrups as their prime ingredients must be avoided as they will cause cravings. The more you eat them, the higher will be the temptation to eat them often.

The same goes for food items with refined flours. Cookies, chips, cakes, candies, bagels, and all other such things are made up of refined flours and sugar. They have a negligible amount of fiber but are high in sugar and carb content. These things will load your system with empty calories but your gut wouldn't get much to process. Such things should also be avoided.

To avoid cravings, try to shift to fresh foods. Eat a lot of fresh fruits and vegetables. If you have a sweet tooth and you want something sweet, you can eat fruit. They have natural sugar that won't lead to cravings. The fruits also have a lot of dietary fiber that provides a lot of material for your gut to process. This is the healthies alternative to harmful sweets.

You can only avoid cravings if you pick the right kind of food products. If you rely too much on processed food items then avoiding sugar may become difficult for you.

# Headaches

When you begin any kind of fasting the most common side-effect that you may feel is a headache. The main reason behind the headaches is the over-reliance of your body on instant sugar refills. When you are eating at frequent intervals, you are also dumping calories at regular intervals. It gets converted into glucose and your body loves to burn it. It is very easy to use fuel. However, when you start observing fasts, your body goes through ketosis and it adjusts itself to burn fat fuel. Fat fuel is comparatively difficult to burn but it provides a lot of energy. But, your body doesn't like to make the switch easily. The headaches are the form of protest your body does.

The good thing is that these headaches are temporary and would go away as soon as your body makes the switch. Once your body starts burning fat for energy, there would be no headaches as it would start getting the required energy effortlessly and without looking at you for it.

If you are feeling headache due to sugar withdrawal symptoms, you can simply have unsweetened black tea or coffee. It will help in suppressing the headache.

# Light-headedness

It is yet another problem that you may face in the initial stages of fasting. There is a very little chance that you keep experiencing it while you adapt yourself to One Meal a Day. It happens as your body notices a change in your eating process and it is battling between lowering the BMR and burning the fat fuel.

It is simply an indication of the fact that ready supply of energy has ended and the body needs you to dump a few calories into the system. If you are feeling lightheaded after getting up or while walking, you must take precautions to avoid accidental falling.

This lightheadedness lasts a couple of days and your body gets adjusted to the fasting schedule.

# Weakness

This shouldn't come as a surprise that you may feel a bit weak in the beginning. However, like all other symptoms, even this is not a permanent thing. While you observe longer fasting hours, your body feels energy deprived and hence there is a feeling of weakness. You shouldn't worry as it would go away as soon as your body starts burning the fat fuel. Our body can run for months without food on the body fat itself. One Meal a Day routine you will be eating 1500-1800 calories a day and hence there is no reason for you to feel weak.

In fact, obesity and associated disorders weaken your body's ability to absorb nutrients from the food you eat. It means that you need to eat a lot more to get even small amounts of nutrients. Your digestive abilities go down. You start getting nutrient deficiencies and have to depend upon nutrient supplements. Eating once a day helps your body and the digestive system in repairing or healing itself. The load on your digestive system goes down and it is able to absorb the nutrients from the food properly. You may also notice that you no longer require nutrient supplements to cure deficiencies.

# Irritation

You may feel irritated at times and that is normal and happens very often when your body is looking for food. Irritation and mood swings are common symptoms. They are also sugar withdrawal symptoms and you don't need to worry about them. Staying away from sugar-rich food items and drinking permitted beverages like black tea or coffee can be of great help in treating the problem.

# Frequent Urination

As we had discussed in the earlier chapters, whenever there will be a calorie deficit, the first thing your body would do is dump a lot of water. It would lead to frequent trips to the washroom. There is nothing to worry about this as it also leads to detoxification and cleansing of the body.

The important thing here is to remember to replenish the loss of fluids. You must drink water whenever thirsty. You must not stall thirst as that can lead to dehydration, headache, irritation, and other such symptoms.

Another important thing to keep in mind is that along with water, there will also be a loss of minerals from your body. This loss can be critical and hence you will have to keep replenishing the minerals. The best way to do that is to mix a pinch of sea salt in the glass of water that you drink. If you are suffering from hypertension, you must not mix salt without consulting your physician.

## Heartburn, Constipation, and Bloating

Heartburn and bloating are common problems in fasting. When you get on any new fasting schedule your gut takes time to adjust. Meanwhile, it keeps releasing the gastric juices at regular intervals that don't get any proper meal to digest. This can lead to a feeling of bloating. The heartburn is also part of the same process. Fortunately, this process is short as your gastric juice release system gets timed automatically very soon and you wouldn't have to face these problems for long.

Some people may also get constipated when getting on a fasting schedule. For them, eating a balanced and fiber-rich diet is the best solution. Such a diet would help in the proper processing of the food and would also ensure good health of the intestinal tract. This way, you can easily get rid of the problem of constipation.

## The Good

One Meal a Day has a lot of benefits and most of the side-effects that you experience in the beginning fade away. It has great positives in store for you.

## High Energy

Once your body switches to fat fuel, you will start feeling a great rush of energy. The fat fuel is clean and produces a negligible amount of toxins and waste material in comparison to glucose fuel. Even a small amount of fat fuel will release a lot of energy. Soon, you would experience that you feel fresh and energetic.

# No Lethargy

The most common feeling after having a meal is lethargy. We all like to sleep a little after having a heavy meal. It happens as the food loads your system with carbs and your blood glucose levels rise steeply. This doesn't happen when your body is burning the fat fuel. It burns at a constant rate and there is minimal production of waste material and toxins. This also helps in avoiding the feeling of lethargy that people experience after meals.

You will always feel energetic and rejuvenated.

# Positive Mood

Glucose fuel causes a lot of mood swings. When your system is loaded with glucose, you may experience joy, however, as soon as your blood glucose levels go down, you start feeling irritation, frustration, and panic. These mood swings can be very troublesome in many people as they are unable to explain the reasons behind their mood swings.

However, that doesn't happen when your body is burning fat fuel through ketosis. The fat fuel releases energy at a consistent rate and hence the probability of mood swings get very low.

# Chapter 16: Setting Goals

Having a clear goal in mind is always very helpful. You can always judge whether you are making progress or not. When it comes to obesity, setting the right goal becomes all the more important as people have an innate fear of failure. Progress keeps them motivated and they are able to give a little extra if they feel they are making headway.

One Meal a Day is a tough routine. It requires a lot of motivation and nothing could motivate a person more than progress. However, setting the right goals is equally important. You must know the areas in which you want to make progress.

There are 3 major goals that people have when taking up One Meal a Day routine:

1. Weight Loss
2. Maintenance of the Current Weight
3. Overall Improvement in Health Biomarkers

# Weight Loss

If you have started One Meal a Day routine for weight loss then you will be pleasantly surprised to find that the success rates are high and the progress is evidently clear from the early stages. Yet, it is important that you look in the right direction. There are two ways in which you can make progress.

    i.     Loss of Weight on Scale

   ii.     Reduction in the Waistline

It comes as a surprise to many that although their waistline recedes while they follow the routine, they may not notice any significant change in their weight on the scale after a certain period.

Does this mean that they have stopped making progress?

The answer is no. They are making good progress but not understanding it clearly. One of the biggest benefits of intermittent fasting methods is that it not only helps you lose weight and burn fat, but it also helps in building muscles. The fat is voluminous and it makes you look bulky although it doesn't weigh much. The muscles are compact but heavy. So, while you are losing fat, you are also building new muscles. Therefore, the chances are that you may not lose much weight on the scale but there will be a significant reduction in the waistline.

Here, it is important to understand that weight is not the actual health problem whereas fat is a problem. So, if you are losing fat and gaining muscles you are making great progress.

You must take both things into account from the very first day. While you weigh yourself on the scale, you must also keep a meticulous record of your waistline to get the correct idea of your progress.

# Maintenance of Current Weight

The biggest problem with obesity is that although you may be able to lose weight maintaining the same for long is tough. This problem is noticed by everyone on any kind of weight loss program. People observe that weight relapse is a very common phenomenon.

One Meal a Day routine is a great program for maintaining your set weight. You will find that maintaining weight has never been easier. If you are following the set routine then the possibility of absurd weight gain is minimal. However, you must maintain a record to keep yourself well-informed and motivated.

# Overall Improvement in Health Biomarkers

In the past few years, there has been a significant improvement in awareness about the dangers posed by a poor lifestyle, bad eating habits, and unhealthy food. It is a remarkable thing. Maintaining and improving health is even better than getting treatment for ailments. As the old adage goes, 'Precaution is better than cure'.

One Meal a Day routine can help you immensely in that area. It is a routine that helps you in keeping blood sugar in check, improves insulin sensitivity, helps in lowering cholesterol, management of blood pressure and several other such issues. However, you can't track most of these things on your own. If you are following the routine for overall improvement in your health biomarkers then you must get a complete health checkup before beginning the routine.

You will also have to get the tests done at regular intervals to assess the progress.

You must mark all your accomplishments without fail as that would give you the push required to keep moving forward. Achieving milestones is the best way to remain motivated on a set path.

# Chapter 17: Risk Factors and Viability of the Routine

All are not created equal in this world. What may be good for one, may not be the same for others. This qualifies for everything in life and even One Meal a Day routine is not an exception. The routine is tough and has some risk factors for people falling under some specific categories. It is important that before beginning the routine you make an assessment whether or not you fall under those categories.

Excellent for Weight Loss But Not So Good for Body Builders

One Meal a Day routine is restrictive in nature. It limits your calorie intake and you may not get all the nutrients required for building muscles like a bodybuilder. If you are simply trying to lose or maintain weight this routine is ideal for you. However, if bodybuilding is your aim, this routine may leave you exasperated. Intermittent fasting routines are excellent for bodybuilding as they boost the production of HGH and adrenaline. Hence, stamina and muscle building gets a great push. However, One Meal a Day routine may fail to provide you the kind of nutrition required for bodybuilding. You can consider other intermittent fasting routines that allow eating a bit more like the warrior fasting routine also known as 20:4 fasting.

People with Pre-existing Medical Conditions Need to Be Cautious

One Meal a Day routine is an excellent program to keep away problems like diabetes, hypertension, and heart problems. However, if you are already suffering from them, things may become a bit different for you. Pre-existing medical conditions put you under risk as you are already under the medication and leaving the medication for such long periods during the fast window can be risky. There is also a risk of blood sugar level fluctuation. If you have such pre-existing conditions then you may not get a level playing field.

In such cases, it is inadvisable for you to begin such fasting without proper medical supervision. You must consult your doctor and then only start the routine.

Pregnant or Lactating Women

The experts have a divided opinion about longer fasting for women. Although they agree on the point that fasting equally helps women as men, some experts believe that longer fasting can mess with the hormonal cycles of women. When it comes to pregnant and lactating women the experts are of the opinion that they shouldn't fast. They have very high nutritional requirements as they are bearing the added responsibility of supporting another life.

# People Suffering from Eating Disorders

If someone is suffering from eating disorders then also following One Meal a Day routine is inadvisable. Such people are already under great stress and stretching it too far can create severe health issues for them.

If you are suffering from any health issue that requires long-term medication, you must not follow this routine without medical advice and supervision. One Meal a Day is a serious commitment and your body may not help you in the routine in such cases.

# Chapter 18: Ways to Get the Most Out of 'One Meal A Day' Routine

One Meal a Day is a great routine and it has immense health benefits. Anyone following the routine properly will get the benefits. However, you may still notice that some people make tremendous progress while others don't have such remarkable success. It is not the fault of the routine but the way they are living up to the routine that creates this difference.

If you want to have success in the routine you will have to understand the needs of your body. The body not only needs to lose weight but it also needs maintenance time. It needs rest as much as it needs exercise. Although fasting is good for you, the right kind of diet can bring a lot of difference in the results.

Given below are the four important things that you must give due attention to have success in your routine:

## A Healthy Diet

Food is an essential requirement of the body. These days, food may have become the prime reason for most of our health problems, yet you can't run this body without food. The kind of food that you eat will always have a profound impact on your progress. We have already discussed that you need to have the right mix of macronutrients for a healthy body.

Fat, protein, and carbs all are equally important in set proportions. Yet, it is important that you understand that every kind of fat is not good for health.

Unsaturated fats can give a boost to your good health whereas saturated fats may increase the risk of heart diseases. The worst are the trans fats that are deadly. You must make an informed decision while choosing the right kind of fat for yourself.

Protein is also important. While you must have the right mix of protein, relying solely on animal protein is not a very good strategy. Nuts and seeds also have high-quality protein. Eggs and dairy also have protein. You can also get good protein from legumes and pulses. Eating the right mix will help you more in staying on the healthy side and experiencing better results.

Carbs are usually portrayed as potential villains. All types of carbs are not bad. While refined carbs or simple carbs are bad as they can spike your blood sugar levels instantly, the complex carbs are very different. Complex carbs are slow to digest and they don't spike your blood sugar levels. Additionally, there are several trace minerals that you can only get through carbs like whole grains and hence avoiding carbs completely can be a very poor strategy.

However, you must always focus on having the right sources of these macronutrients in the ideal proportions to get the best health benefits.

# Exercise

Exercise is essential to get the benefits of One Meal a Day. It is a way to force your body to burn those extra calories that would make the difference in your weight and obesity.

Some people may not be in a position to follow a strict exercise routine due to their weight and work routines. Yet, nothing can stop them from being active in their daily life. A sedentary lifestyle is among the prime reasons for obesity and you can't fight it by sitting idle or doing nothing extra.

The intensity of your exercise routine will determine the speed of your weight loss. However, for those who aren't in a position to do intense exercises, they also must do light exercise. Walking, jogging, swimming, yoga, aerobic exercises are some of the routines that can be followed easily. Even if you have excess weight, walking every day is possible. Even if you have a traveling job and hitting the gym daily isn't possible for you, a few squats in your hotel room are easily possible.

One Meal a Day routine will create the right conditions to lose weight. You can capitalize on it by adding exercise to your daily routine. You must never ignore the exercise routine and should always involve some kind of exercise in your daily life.

High-intensity interval training (HIIT) is usually the best routine to lose weight. You need to perform some intense exercises in short intervals. This puts pressure on specific regions and has an excellent impact on your weight loss. You can perform HIIT on alternate days and do light exercises on the resting days.

The important thing is to bring exercise into your life and increase its duration gradually.

# <u>Sleep</u>

Sleep is equally important for your health if not more. It is the time your body needs for making a full recovery and doing the repair work. If you want good health you can't ignore sleep. You must give yourself ample time to rest and recover.

The current lifestyle has become very hectic. There are deadlines, competition, worries, stress, and fear that has stolen our peaceful sleep time. Whatever was left of it was snatched away by social media and the smartphones. The first thing that we try to look for in the morning is our smartphone. The last thing we have a look at before going to sleep is again the smartphone. It has the power to push your sleep aside for hours. It is eating our personal time yet there is nothing much we can do about it. However, to stay healthy and fit, it is important that you don't compromise on your sleep time.

It is during your sleep that most essential fat burning hormones are produced. It is during your sleep time that your body is able to repair the damage incurred during the day.

One of the biggest side-effects is also problems with sleeping. Sleep apnea is a reality known to most people facing obesity. However, mixing the right kind of diet and exercise can help you in getting good sleep.

# Lifestyle

Our lifestyle also has a very important role to play in our health. Losing weight has a lot to do with a positive attitude. If your attitude is not positive, you may not get the desired results. Our lifestyles have become such that the scope of staying positive has gone down drastically.

We begin our days with a frown. We are always stressed about family, deadlines, competition, finance, economy, politics, society, our neighbors and what not. The problem is that in most of these things we do not have a direct control yet we are stressing ourselves with the tension and that is ruining our health.

We have stopped treating the day as day and night as night. We don't find it odd to sleep till late in the day or remain awake partying or watching TV till late at night. We are messing with the circadian rhythm of nature. This also puts a lot of strain on the body and contributes heavily to weight gain.

If you want to get the full benefits of One Meal a Day routine you will have to ensure improvement in your lifestyle. It doesn't require much. You will simply need to give your body the required rest. Stop playing by hectic deadlines. Ensure that you maintain a reasonably active lifestyle and enjoy your life as much as you can.

Bringing positivity into your lifestyle can be very helpful in bringing down your weight. The more you feel crumbled down by weight the tougher it will get to get over it.

# Chapter 19: Impact of Water and Juice Fasting on Weight Loss

There are several ways in which you can try to improve the results of your fasting. You can expand the benefits with water and juice fasting. The concept is as simple as it sounds. You will simply have to remove the meal and replace it with water or fruits and vegetable blends.

## Juice Fasting

It is a popular concept these days and people are following it in droves. You can simply blend the fruits and vegetables and drink them. Juicing them is not very advisable as it takes out all the fiber from them and you only get the juice which can spike your blood sugar levels. Juice fasting is something that you can do occasionally for 2-3 days. Doing it for longer than this might not have additional health benefits. However, you must also remember that you will have to remain extra careful while getting off your juice fast. 2-3 days of food deprivation calls for slow progression to solid food. This means that the next day you cannot begin with solid food. You will have to start with soups and then follow up with semi-solid food and eventually solid food. Not following this precaution can have an adverse health impact.

Juice fasting has become very popular as it is very easy to do and has good weight loss benefits. People are going after it with great enthusiasm.

There are some common reasons for doing so:

Fruits and Vegetables are Full of Antioxidants and Phytonutrients

It is a well-known fact that fruits and vegetables are full of antioxidants and phytonutrients. They help your body in fighting chronic inflammations. Fruits and vegetables are also high in vitamins and minerals and hence they help in providing extra nutrients and boosting overall health. Their anti-inflammatory properties help in boosting your immune system and you will start feeling more energetic.

## They are Low in Calories

Fruits and vegetables are low in calories. You can bring your calorie intake to half by following a juice fast. So, if you want to follow a calorie conscious routine for a few days you can do juice fasting.

## They Help in Detoxification of the Body

It is popularly believed that juices help in clearing out toxins from the body. Although studies have not been able to substantiate this fact.

## They are good for Your Gut

It is a fact that juice fasting can help in improving your gut health. There are several healthy enzymes in fruits and vegetables that help in improving your digestive system. So, you can expect your digestion system to work more efficiently after this fasting.

Some Important Things to Note

- Drinking juices in large quantities carry some risks. Certain juices contain oxalate which can cause the formation of kidney stones.
- Too much juice can also cause diarrhea. This means that you will be at risk of losing too many nutrients and may experience weakness.
- It can also cause an imbalance in electrolytes and you may start experiencing dehydration.

# Water Fasting

Water fasting is a very common and safe way to fast. The biggest benefit of water fasting is that it helps in kick-starting autophagy. This single benefit can outsmart any other benefit. When you are doing water fasting there is no intake of calories. Your body experiences a complete energy cut-off and it starts the process of running the body more efficiently to conserve the energy for the longest periods. This means that it will become a chronic inflammation fighting machine and a recycler.

You can do water fasting once a month for 2-3 days. Don't do water fasting longer than that as it may lower your metabolism. For the first few days, your body remains in an alert condition so that it can get food. However, when it doesn't get food for longer than 72 hours, the starvation mode kicks in. In this mode, the metabolic rate goes very low to conserve as much energy as possible and your body's main concern becomes survival. There will not be any significant weight loss in this stage and you may experience severe weakness.

Apart from Autophagy some of the benefits of water fasting are:

It Helps in Bringing Down Blood Pressure

Water fasting has a great impact on your blood pressure. People with high blood pressure experience a severe drop in their blood pressure. One of the main reasons behind this is the absence of salt intake during these fasts.

## **Lowers Oxidative Stress**

Poor food choice and unhealthy lifestyle lead to a lot of oxidative stress on your body. This oxidative stress is responsible for causing several types of chronic inflammations. Too much accumulation of reactive oxygen species (ROS) takes place in your body. Water fasting helps in flushing out these ROS from your body.

Improves Leptin and Insulin Sensitivity

Insulin sensitivity will automatically improve when you keep the insulin release under check in your body. This happens on its own in water fasting as you will not be consuming anything with calories. The same goes for leptin. Your brain becomes more sensitive to this satiety hormone when you get off food for an extended period.

Although water fasting is good for your health, you must remember that getting off the water fasting is as important as the fast. Like juice fasting, you will not be able to eat solid food immediately after getting off the water fasting. You must start with liquids then move on to semi-solid food and finally eat solid food. This process helps your gut in adjusting to the change.

# Chapter 20: Understanding the Risk of overhydration

Someone who has been on a fast ever will surely understand the importance of water in fasting. Apart from the health benefits, it is the only thing that really helps in suppressing the hunger pangs. You can fill your tummy with water and divert your attention from food for a bit longer.

The world praises water but no one talks about the risks of overhydration although it is equally dangerous as dehydration.

## How Does Over hydration Occur?

Over hydration occurs when you start drinking more water than needed. Water is essential but your body doesn't like to keep anything that's not required. If you are drinking too much water then your body will have to pump it out in the form of urine and it would be an extra load. Besides that, when you are drinking more water you will also have to pee a lot. Along with the water body also starts losing a lot of minerals too. It can cause electrolyte imbalance.

## What is the Effect of overhydration?

The job of cleaning waste from the body is of kidneys. So, if you start drinking a lot of water, it would put a lot of strain on them without reason. Overhydration occurs when you start drinking more water than your kidneys can process. This is not very healthy.

## How to check for overhydration?

Keep a look at the color of your urine. If your urine is dark yellow, it means that you are dehydrated. However, when the color of the urine is like water it means you are drinking copious amounts of water and you must control your water intake.

## How Much Water Should We Drink?

You should only drink when you feel thirsty. Don't drink water because others have told you or because you haven't had water for long. Drink it when you feel thirsty and you wouldn't have to worry about it. The water intake would naturally increase when you are doing some labor intensive job like exercise or in summers. However, drinking water for the sake of it should be avoided.

When you begin fasting your water intake would increase as you wouldn't be eating anything and it helps in struggling with hunger but it shouldn't be used in excess.

# Chapter 21: One Meal a Day Routine on Keto Diet

Some people believe that all the calories are the same. However, that's not true. When you eat a carbohydrate-rich diet, it releases a lot of glucose instantly but this energy is short lived. Your body would start processing it fast as it needs to lower the blood sugar levels and you would start feeling hungry very soon. Fat and protein-rich diet, on the other hand, is very dense and releases energy very slowly. This is what helps you in going without food for longer. Fat and protein-rich diets are known as a keto diet.

Before we proceed further it is important to understand the process of ketosis as the reference would come time and again.

## Ketosis

Ketosis is the process of where your body begins to burn fat in place of carbohydrates. It is a very important process required for burning the fat in your body too.

Our body is an engine that runs on fuel like any other machine. It has the ability to run on two types of fuel, glucose fuel, and fat fuel. When you eat carbs it releases a lot of glucose into your bloodstream. The insulin is dumped into the system by the pancreas to stabilize the blood sugar levels. Insulin is a fat-storage hormone and hence until there is insulin in your blood, the body would never enter the fat burning mode.

The ketogenic diet or keto diet is fat and protein-rich diet and it has very little to no carbs. This means that your body stops getting glucose to burn for energy and hence it switches to fat burning. The fat is slow to digest and hence there is no energy spike and your body keeps functioning smoothly.

When there is no glucose supply from outside the body has no other option than to metabolize fat. The liver produces hormones that start breaking the fat cells.

# How to Begin Ketosis?

There are three main ways to begin ketosis.

By Reducing Carb Intake

The Keto diets are rich in fat and proteins. They have very low carb content and the carbs are also complex carbs that are slow to break. This means that the body stops getting a ready supply of glucose and it has no other option than to burn fatty acids. The liver releases ketones that break the fatty acids and produces energy.

By Doing Intense Physical Exercise

When you do intense physical exercise, your body burns the glucose fuel aggressively and soon your glucose stores get low. Then it starts breaking glycogen stores and eventually there is no other option left other than using fatty acids for producing energy.

By Fasting

Fasting is also a good way to induce ketosis. The glucose lasts only for a few hours and the body has to begin using the glycogen stores for producing energy. However, if you remain in the fasted state for longer than 20 hours, the glycogen stores also don't last and the body has to begin burning fatty acids for energy.

## **One Meal a Day Routine on Keto Diet**

One Meal a Day routine on a keto diet is a great way to push your body into ketosis. Your body already remains in a fasted state for very long. The absence of carbs in your diet ensures that your body only gets fat and protein for burning. This is the same fuel as the fatty acids and hence remaining in a ketosis state gets easier for the body as it doesn't have to switch fuel types time and again.

If you want to lose weight, following a keto diet with One Meal a Day routine will be the most helpful.

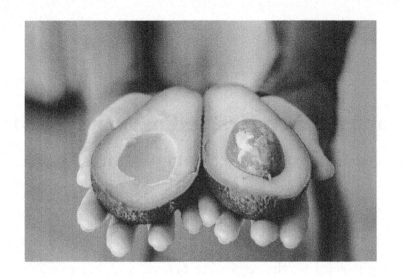

# Part IV

## Chapter 22: Understanding Popular Myths and Why Not to Worry About Them

There are several myths regarding fasting and most of them don't have any scientific basis. It is important that you understand them and the reasons for not to worry about them.

### Myth #1 Fasting Triggers Starvation Mode

This is a very popular myth for unknown reasons. I believe that people who have a phobia of staying hungry for long have popularized this concept. The people who say this have no understanding of the starvation mode and the way our body functions.

When you stay without food for an extended period, your body begins to sense the urgency of food. It knows that you need to be more alert and active to get food and hence your reflexes improve. Imagine starvation mode kicking on our ancestors. They would have perished away and we wouldn't have seen the light of day. Finding food was a challenge for them as they were facing extreme odds. The beasts they were trying to catch were much better than them in all respects. The animals they hunted were faster, had better powers of hearing and smell. They also had stronger and longer teeth and nails. If staying without food for a day could kick starvation mode, our ancestors might not have been able to get the next meal ever.

On the contrary, the body increases the reflexes after a few hours of fasting so that you can function better to get food. The starvation mode is a reality. However, it only kicks in after you have gone without food for around 90 hours. By this time the body starts conserving the energy to wait for the favorable times when you can get a resupply of energy.

Fasting is generally practiced for shorter durations and hence there is no danger of starvation mode kicking in.

## Myth #2 Fasting Slows Down Your Metabolism

This is again a myth made popular by food production industry which wants you to keep eating due to its vested interests. They believe that if we stop eating for a few hours our metabolism will slow down. We have a very robust metabolic system. It cannot slow down if you don't eat for a few hours.

If you follow calorie restrictive diets, there is a danger of metabolism slowing down as the body starts noticing the lower intake of food.

However, if you remain in a fasted state and you eat normally in the eating windows, no such change would get noticed as the body would be switching to fat burning to fulfill its energy needs. Studies have shown that during the fasting periods, your metabolism increases by 14%.

## Myth #3 Fasting Leads to Muscle Loss

People believe that if they don't eat food, the body will start cannibalizing itself and eat all the muscles. This myth has come into existence based on the knowledge that our body can use excess protein for producing energy.

It is true that if you eat excess protein than required your body breaks it down to produce energy. However, there is no truth behind the fact that it would start eating its own active muscles for producing energy.

On the contrary, studies have demonstrated that fasting leads to the production of hormones that help in building muscles.

## Myth #4 Fasting Will Make You Feel Extremely Hungry All the Time

No, fasting will not make you feel extremely hungry all the time. Hunger pangs are a result of the release of a hunger hormone called ghrelin. Our gut releases this hormone periodically to indicate the brain that food should be consumed. However, if you suppress your hunger for a bit long the ghrelin levels go down and you stop feeling hungry.

Your hunger pangs would also depend upon the kind of food you are consuming in your eating window. Consumption of a carb-rich diet will make you hungry fast as it gets processed quickly. However, the same is not true for fat and protein-rich diet as it takes much longer to process this dense diet.

## Myth #5 Fasting Increases Stress Hormone Cortisol

Cortisol is the stress hormone that has several functions in our body. It is responsible for maintaining blood pressure, regulating the immune system and breaking down of proteins, glucose, and lipids. Cortisol levels in our body may increase on several occasions and that may not have any negative impact.

When you do the aggressive physical activity your body produces cortisol. It helps in the metabolization of fat for producing energy. It also increases your performance. Fasting also leads to a minor increase in the cortisol levels but that only induces positive stress on your body. It doesn't have any negative impact.

If you are morbidly obese that would lead to the creation of extreme stress on the body and it would produce cortisol. In such conditions, it starts acting against your body as it senses the distress and stops the fat burning activity.

# Chapter 23: Staying Motivated

One of the most important things on a weight loss journey is to stay motivated throughout the way. Weight loss is never easy and people trying to lose weight are already under great pressure. They take the flak from their peers, friends, and family and want to get rid of the problem as fast as possible. This desperation to get rid of the problem makes them impatient. However, losing weight and keeping it under check requires a lot of patience and perseverance.

One Meal a Day routine is also not a very easy program and hence people may get demotivated very fast. It is important that you always have the goal in front of you and keep working towards it. Being impatient will only bring more miseries to you.

Obesity is not just a cosmetic problem that you need to resolve to look presentable in society. It is much deeper and has far-reaching consequences. It has profound physiological as well as psychological effects. The more weight one has the more difficult it gets to shed it. This makes the impatience highly risky.

If you don't have your support firmly grounded, bearing the same can get even more difficult. It is important that you always remain grounded and firm. Weight loss is a consequence of the process and would happen eventually. Your focus should always remain on getting rid of the problems that have caused the excess weight to accumulate.

Remaining positive is the only way through which you can avoid problems. You need to hold your ground and keep moving toward your goal.

To bear the pressure of facing others and coming out of the feelings of self-doubt, you can do the following things.

## Use Positive Affirmations

Listening to positive affirmations, reciting and believing on them is a great way to get over the feelings of self-doubt. There are thousands of books on positive affirmations, videos on the internet that can help you. You must make use of them to remain positive.

## Discuss It with Your Trusted and Loved Ones

Friends and family can always prove to be your strongest support. One Meal a Day can be a very demanding routine. There will be times when you may feel like dropping it. There would be times when you may feel tempted to eat. There can also be times when you wouldn't feel satisfied with the results and would want to throw the towel. However, if you have confided in your friends and family members, they can provide the required moral support. They can also help in many other ways like not eating carelessly when you are around or not displaying food in your fasting window. The same goes for your friends. One of the biggest reasons for binge eating or unwanted eating is the persistence of friends. If you disclose your routine or about your weight loss efforts they would understand it and wouldn't create situations in which you have to make a tough choice.

## Professional Help

You can also take the help of health professionals in your health goals. A health professional will be able to guide you according to your needs and also keep a close watch on your progress. This is also very helpful when you are also battling with some pre-existing illness and need supervision in your fasting. A professional can provide you moral as well as medical support for all your needs.

## Support Groups

Joining a support group is another way to remain motivated. Support groups have individuals suffering from similar issues and they share their problems and success stories. You will also be able to know about the challenges others have faced and the way they have overcome those problems. They can give you an exact idea of situations to come and the ways to avoid unpleasant things in the way. Above all, they lend you the ears without being judgmental so that you can open your heart and feel light.

## Make Your Home More Fasting Friendly

Strongest resolves break in the weakest moments when you are the most vulnerable. These are the times when you are not able to follow restraint. Hunger can create such moments and the best way to avoid them is to keep your fridge and kitchen free of such things that can tempt you into eating. Keeping sodas, chips, fries and other ready to eat things away is also a great idea. Don't keep your fridge stuffed with such things as that can lead to temptation every time you open the fridge even for drinking water.

Keep a Keen Eye on Your Progress and Celebrate Even Smaller Victories

The life is not all about bigger victories, the smaller ones keep refueling you with vigor. You must keep a close watch on your progress and celebrate even small milestones that you achieve. In that way, it would be easier for you to maintain control.

In the end, it is all about you. You are going to be the biggest and sole beneficiary of your efforts. Obesity is restrictive in nature. It limits the possibilities for you. There are many opportunities that slip from your hand because you may not find yourself in a position to grab them due to your condition. One Meal a Day routine can help you in overcoming these limitations. All you need to do is hang on for a little more and keep doing what you are doing.

# Conclusion

Thanks for making it through to the end of this book, let's hope it was informative and able to provide you with all of the tools you need to achieve your goals whatever they may be.

One Meal A Day routine is a powerful technique to shed the extra weight and bring your fat under control. It is a systematic process through which you can easily lead a healthy and fit life.

This book has tried to explain not only the basics of One Meal a Day routine but also the correct way to incorporate it into your life. The key to success in this routine is to remain patient and follow the steps correctly. You must not rush the process and always keep the basics in mind.

Following quick fixes for losing weight may give you results in the short-term but they can never last long and such methods have their own side-effects. One Meal a Day routine is safe, reliable and very effective. You only need to follow it with patience and perseverance.

You can also get all the benefits of the process by following the simple steps given in the book. I hope that this book is really able to help you in achieving your health goals.

Finally, if you found this book useful in any way, a review on Amazon is always appreciated!

Made in the USA
Monee, IL
09 February 2021